Teen Brains & HIV: Balancing Meds & Development

Sachin

First Printing, 2024

Table of Contents

Introduction

Since the roll out of antiretroviral therapy (ART), the treatment for Human Immunodeficiency Virus/Acquired Immunodeficiency Syndrome (HIV/AIDS), in 2005, South Africa has realized major turnarounds in the course of HIV/AIDS, including reduced HIV-related morbidity and mortality rates (Statistics South Africa, 2019). However, despite an increase in the roll out of ART, HIV/AIDS remains a key national public health concern in South Africa (Global AIDS monitoring, 2018). In keeping with the global target of eradicating HIV/AIDS by 2030, the South African government took critical policy decisions aimed at combating the HIV/AIDS pandemic; ensuring, for example, that ART is available at public health service points (Statistics South Africa, 2019). The decision to roll out ART within the public health sector has produced significant gains; evidenced mainly by extended life spans of people living with HIV, for all affected ages (Statistics South Africa, 2019). However, poor adherence to ART threatens to reverse these gains. Generally, inconsistencies in adherence to ART have been identified as one of the leading contributors to ART failure (Falagas, Zarkadoulia, Pliatsika, & Panos, 2008; Giacomet et al., 2003; Solomon & Halkitis, 2008) and has been noted to be particularly problematic amongst adolescents. Commonly, it is during adolescence that individuals typically learn of their HIV-positive status (Smith & Wilkins, 2015; Wiener, Mellins, Marhefka, & Battles, 2007) and also the stage where the responsibility of taking ART transfers from primary caregivers to personal responsibility (Giacomet et al., 2003; Smith & Wilkins, 2015).

Of note, poor adherence to ART in adolescents has been identified as a key contributing factor to the persistence of some forms of neurocognitive impairment (Cattie, Doyle, Weber, Grant, & Woods, 2012; Hermetet-Lindsay et al., 2017). Specifically, there is growing evidence in research of greater prevalence of executive function impairments in HIV-positive adolescents than previously acknowledged (Cattie et al., 2012; Clark et al., 2017; Laughton et al., 2013). Executive function generally refers to goal directed behaviour (Diamond, 2013). Impairment in this domain commonly results in every day functional decline and research suggests that it can also contribute to poor adherence patterns to ART (Diamond, 2013; Wood, Shah, Steenhoff, & Rutstein, 2009). Studies further show that executive dysfunction can directly impact adherence to ART particularly in adolescents, where continued brain development, especially in the frontal lobes, takes place (Kim et al., 2014; Laughton et al., 2013; Nichols et al., 2016).

However, studies on executive functions and individuals with HIV are typically conducted on adult populations, and there is limited data on paediatric populations, particularly from South Africa (Laughton et al., 2013; Nichols et al., 2016). Given the necessity of good adherence for optimal health among HIV-positive adolescents, and the role that executive functions might contribute in achieving that goal, investigations into executive functioning generally, and in relation to adherence within the adolescent population, is pertinent.

Literature Review

Human Immunodeficiency Virus/Acquired Immunodeficiency Syndrome (HIV/AIDS)

HIV is the virus that causes AIDS and is classified as a lentivirus. Two types of HIV are commonly reported in literature, HIV-1 and HIV-2 (Nyamweya et al., 2013). HIV-1 is more prevalent worldwide with HIV-2 more endemic in West Africa and in some parts of India (Nyamweya et al., 2013). Besides genome and geographic differences, these HIV types also differ in rates of infectivity or rates of transmission, with HIV-1 having a comparatively higher rate of transmission than HIV-2 (Esbjörnsson et al., 2019; Nyamweya et al., 2013). Another key difference is that with HIV-2 immunodeficiency occurs at a much slower rate, however, the life expectancy of those with HIV-2 is shorter than those with HIV-1 (Esbjörnsson et al., 2019; Nyamweya et al., 2013). HIV-1 infection, which is more prominent in Southern Africa, can be categorized into four main groups: M, N, O, P. Most HIV infections worldwide derive from group M; within this group 12 subtypes/clades are identified (subtype A – L). In South Africa, specifically, HIV-1 clade C is the most prevalent HIV infection subtype (Jacobs et al., 2009; Joska et al., 2011; Santos & Soares, 2010).

HIV epidemiology. By the end of 2018, approximately 37.9 million people worldwide were living with HIV (WHO, 2019). Additionally, in 2018 it was estimated that 770 000 people died from HIV-related causes and that there were 1.7 million new infections (WHO, 2019). However, despite these high figures, recent global data on the incidence of HIV reflects improvements in trends overtime. For example, global annual AIDS-related deaths, have declined from 1.9 million in 2004 to 940 000 in 2017 (UNAIDS, 2018). Global estimates further showed a decline in new infections, from 3.4 to 1.8 million, from 1996 to 2017, respectively (UNAIDS, 2018). Global reductions in AIDS-related mortality rates were mainly attributed to increases in the rollout of HIV/AIDS treatment services (UNAIDS, 2018). However, even with these promising estimates, it is reported that 180 000 children globally were infected with HIV in 2017, and in the same year, only 50% of HIV-infected children under the age of 15 were receiving treatment (UNAIDS, 2018). Hence, there is still much work to be done among youth with HIV.

Notwithstanding recent downward global trends of several key HIV indices, Sub-Saharan Africa (SSA) remains deeply affected by the HIV/AIDS pandemic. To illustrate, of the estimated 37.9 million people worldwide living with HIV in 2017, 19.6 million were from SSA, specifically, Eastern and Southern Africa (UNAIDS, 2018). It is reported that in 2017 not only did SSA make up 53% of the world's HIV population, but that 45% of global new infections were from countries within SSA (UNAIDS, 2018). For example, in 2017 alone, 800 000 people (650 000 - 1 000 000) were infected with HIV in SSA making this region a hotspot for the virus (UNAIDS, 2018). Consistent with global HIV/AIDS estimates, key HIV/AIDS indicators for the SSA also reflect a downward trend. For instance, AIDS-related deaths in SSA declined by 42% and estimates for new infections overtime show a 30% decline from 2010 to 2017 (UNAIDS, 2018). The regional reduction in AIDS-related mortality rates was mainly attributed to an increased rollout of HIV/AIDS treatment services (UNAIDS, 2018).

In South Africa, a regional analysis in 2017 revealed that the country was among those with the highest incidence of HIV in Sub-Saharan Africa (UNAIDS, 2018). Further, the national HIV prevalence rate in 2018 stood at 13.1% (Statistics South Africa, 2018). According to UNAIDS (2018) in 2017 in South Africa, 280 000 children below the age of fourteen were living with HIV. Also consistent with global and regional trends, South Africa's national HIV-related mortality rates also appear to be steadily declining over time. Specifically, the number of AIDS-related deaths has decreased steadily over time from 267 417 in 2007 to 126 805 in 2019. Again, the observed decline in AIDS-related deaths was attributed to wider access to ART from increased and wider provincial roll out of ART especially within the public health sector (Statistics South Africa, 2019).

HIV transmission. Children commonly contract HIV vertically (i.e., from mother to child, either in-utero, during birth or through breastfeeding (Hoare et al., 2016). Hence, a number of adolescents have lived with HIV since birth. However, the introduction of ARV treatment to pregnant mothers has resulted in a marked decline in prenatal transmission of HIV (Smith & Wilkins, 2015). Other transmission modes of HIV infection, commonly reported among adolescents, are more behavioural, i.e., through sexual contact, blood transfusions and use of contaminated drug instruments (Nagarajan et al., 2012).

HIV pathophysiology. HIV enters the central nervous system (CNS) relatively early in the disease process by crossing the blood brain barrier (BBB) (Chiriboga, Fleishman, Champion, Gaye-Robinson, & Abrams, 2005; Kumar et al., 2009; McArthur, Brew, & Nath, 2005). The BBB is a protective layer of endothelial cells surrounding the CNS separating it from the rest of the body (Abbott, Rönnbäck, & Hansson, 2006). The BBB is highly selective in what it allows into the brain and excludes potentially harmful substances to the brain (Abbot et al., 2006). Amongst its functions, the BBB is responsible for regulating the environment within the brain, ensuring that the environment is conducive for optimum neuronal signalling (Abbot et al., 2006). However, despite the efficacy of the BBB as a protective barrier, the HI virus is able to penetrate it and manages to cross into the CNS within weeks of infection through infected monocytes, macrophages, and lymphocytes, which are able to cross the BBB unimpeded (Abbot et al., 2006; Chiriboga et al., 2005; Koekkoek, de Sonneville, Wolfs, Licht, & Geelen, 2008; Llorente et al., 2014; McArthur et al., 2005; Tan & McArthur, 2012; Van Rie, Harrington, Dow, & Robertson, 2007).

Once in the brain HIV replicates itself and triggers extensive neurotoxic effects and acute inflammatory processes which activate the production of cytokines, which are proteins that assist in the regulation of immune cells to sites of infection (Smith & Wilkins, 2015; WHO, 2019). The secondary inflammatory and neurotoxic processes incite massive depletion of CD4 cells, which are responsible for fighting infections in the body; these processes further promote damage to synaptic-dendritic networks and ultimately bring about widespread destruction of neurons (Sarma et al., 2014; Smith & Wilkins, 2015; Tan & McArthur, 2012; Thomas, Greenfield, Talavera, & Roos, 2016; Van Rie, Harrington, Dow, & Robertson, 2007). The chronic inflammatory and neurotoxicity processes are also implicated in added weakening of the BBB, which fosters further entry of the HI virus into the CNS. Eventually, due to prolonged activation, the immune system becomes compromised to the point of being effectively defenceless against opportunistic diseases (Nyamweya et al., 2013; Smith & Wilkins, 2015; WHO, 2019).

Key brain regions affected by HIV. Although HIV has widespread impact on the brain and is generally known to be regionally nonspecific (Chiriboga et al., 2005, Mitchell, 2006), some studies suggest that damage to the basal ganglia is the hallmark of HIV, and that this neuroanatomical structure is especially vulnerable to HIV infection (Laughton et al., 2013; McArthur et al., 2005; Woods, Moore, Weber, & Grant, 2009). Other brain regions that are particularly vulnerable to HIV include the brain stem, the frontal cortex and deep white matter (Abbott et al., 2006; Laughton et al., 2013; Smith & Wilkins, 2015; Thomas et al., 2016). Woods et al. (2009) also note that HIV has a predilection for the fronto-striatal pathways; however, this apparent predilection may be mediated by damage to the basal ganglia. Combined evidence from neuroimaging studies of both infected adolescents and adults further point out that HIV affects the anatomical structure and function of white matter tracts and numerous neural networks and various brain regions including temporal, parietal cortices and the brain stem (P. Anderson, 2002; McArthur et al., 2005; Sarma et al., 2014). The suggestion that HIV is partial to frontal cortices including frontal circuitries and deep white matter may well explain the presentation of EF deficits seen in HIV-positive individuals, including adolescents. In support of the viewpoint that HIV preferentially affects the frontal regions of the brain, Spies et al. (2016) reports that an HIV diagnosis particularly in childhood is linked to morphological and functional alterations in the frontal brain regions, which are associated with poor neuropsychological outcomes.

For example, a study by Sarma et al. (2014), using magnetic resonance imaging (MRI) to compare the brain scans of prenatally-infected adolescents on ART ($N = 16$) (one adolescent contracted HIV through a blood transfusion before age 1) and aged-matched Controls ($N = 14$), found marked differences in white matter and grey matter volumes between the two groups. Essentially, the study found bilateral white matter atrophy predominantly in the corpus callosum and external capsule and grey matter hypertrophy in various brain areas (including frontal, occipital and temporal gyri) in the brain images of the HIV-positive group relative to the controls. The authors attributed the white matter loss to HIV-related neural injury and death caused by axonal disconnections. The study further observed grey matter volume increase in the HIV- positive adolescents' brain scans. The authors noted that this was an unexpected finding and postulated that the grey matter increase was likely attributable to HIV-related chronic inflammation in the brain as well as probable toxicity from ART, both which may have resulted in swelling of neurons.

Another study by Cohen et al. (2015) of 35 HIV-positive adolescents and 37 HIV-negative controls aged 8 - 18 years also found significant differences in white matter and grey matter volumes. Even though the sample was virologically suppressed and generally clinically asymptomatic (28 of the HIV-positive group were on ART), the study noted lower brain volumes for the HIV-positive group. In this instance, the white and grey matter in the HIV-positive group was smaller in comparison to the controls. The study findings further noted diffuse white matter hyper-intensities in the HIV-positive group suggestive of ongoing immune activation and specifically indicative of gliosis, myelin loss or vascular injury.

Collectively, the findings of the above-mentioned studies highlight potential changes in brain morphology from HIV infection, as well as the likely long-term effects of HIV, even in the context of ART treatment in some studies. Given these brain morphological changes, there exists vast literature on the neurocognitive disorders associated with HIV infection.

Neurocognitive disorders among individuals living with HIV. HIV is associated with moderate to severe neurocognitive impairments, even in the context of increased access to HIV treatment (Donald et al., 2015; Van Rie et al., 2007). These impairments are commonly referred to as HIV associated neurocognitive disorders (HAND) (Heaton et al., 2011; Laughton et al., 2016).

HIV associated neurocognitive disorders (HAND). Researchers have reported that an estimated 30-60% of HIV-positive individuals have some degree of HAND (Cattie et al., 2012; Cross, Combrinck, & Joska, 2013; Wagner at al., 2016). HAND generally affects several cognitive domains (Woods et al., 2009). The taxonomy of HAND includes Asymptomatic neurocognitive impairment (ANI), Mild neurocognitive disorder (MND) and HIV- associated dementia (HAD) (Antinori, Heaton, & Marder, 2007; McArthur et al., 2005; Woods et al., 2009).

Asymptomatic neurocognitive impairment (ANI). A diagnosis of ANI requires neurocognitive impairment in at least two domains without, however, interference in activities of daily living (ADLs). There should also be no delirium or signs of dementia.

Mild neurocognitive disorder (MND). HIV-associated MND is similarly characterized by impairment in two or more neurocognitive domains, however there is mild interference in ADLs in this classification. Neurocognitive impairment in this classification should not meet criteria for dementia or delirium.

HIV associated dementia (HAD). HAD encompasses moderate to severe neurocognitive impairment typically in multiple domains with marked interference in ADLs.

Based on their recent research on HIV-positive adolescents, with the recognition that the distinction between the different categories can be marginal, Hoare et al. (2016) proposed a revised taxonomy of HAND, in which the main point of departure is the inclusion of functional competence when determining the degree of impairment. In this taxonomy, HIV-positive adolescents were classified along four types: no impairment, asymptomatic neurocognitive impairment, minor neurocognitive impairment and major neurocognitive impairment. A diagnosis for major neurocognitive impairment is given when the score on the Child Behaviour Checklist (CBCL) is <35, over and above impairment in two cognitive domains (Hoare et al., 2016).

HIV encephalopathy (HIVE). HIVE is the most severe form of HAND and is considered to be one of the most common CNS neurologic presentations of HIV infection in children and adolescents (Donald et al., 2015). HIVE refers to generalized brain disease and damage associated with HIV (Donald et al., 2015; Mitchell, 2006). Brain scans of individuals with HIVE show diffuse cortical atrophy and widespread symmetrical deep white matter lesions (MacArthur et al., 2005). Fortunately, the introduction of HIV treatment (ART) has curbed the incidence of HIVE (McArthur et al., 2005).

Neuropsychological Presentation of HIV. As noted, HAND generally affects a number of neurocognitive domains (Woods et al., 2009). A neuropsychological profile of

HIV-positive adolescents is therefore broad and generally includes deficits in general intellectual functioning, learning, attention, information processing speed, motor abilities, episodic memory, visual spatial ability and executive function (Fellows et al., 2014; Heaton et al., 2011; Heaton et al., 2015; Koekkoek et al., 2008; Nichols et al., 2016; Ruel et al., 2012; Woods et al., 2009). However, this study focusses primarily on general intellectual functioning and executive function, discussed below.

General intellectual functioning. Significant disparities have been noted in intellectual functioning between HIV-positive adolescents and controls, with HIV-positive adolescents obtaining lower IQ scores than their control counterparts (Cohen et al., 2015; Koekkoek et al., 2008). Additionally, HIV-positive adolescents are more inclined to present with memory and learning difficulties when compared to samples of matched HIV-negative adolescents, which may impact on general intellectual functioning (Nichols et al., 2016; Wood, Shah, Steenhoff, & Rutstein, 2009). A study by Cohen et al. (2015) of HIV-positive adolescents ($n = 35$) and HIV-negative controls ($n = 37$) established that the HIV-positive cohort performed comparatively poorly on tests of IQ than the controls. Similarly, a study by (Hoare et al. (2016), which assessed a sample of South African children and adolescents (age 6 -16), found that comparatively, HIV-positive children and adolescents ($n = 86$) performed more poorly than HIV-negative matched controls ($n = 34$) on verbal and performance IQ subtests.

Executive functions (EF). Executive function is a multifaceted neuropsychological construct that entails a diverse range of mental processes which include planning, decision making, self-regulation, processing information, inhibition of inappropriate behaviours, problem solving and sequencing and monitoring behaviour (Diamond, 2013; Nichols et al., 2016; Nyongesa et al., 2019; Wood, Shah, Steenhoff, & Rutstein, 2009). For this reason, executive functions impact several aspects of living such as academic performance, psychological development, general social interaction and vocational prospects (Diamond, 2013). Given the multifactorial nature of executive function it is not surprising that they have an overarching reach over quality of life and that such deficits are more likely to impair the capacity to undertake everyday tasks effectively and can degenerate to general functional decline.

Given that executive functions are broad and multifactorial in nature, evaluating them through the rubric of a model is helpful; in this study I used P. Anderson's executive function model.

Executive function model. P. Anderson (2002) proposes a model that provides an insightful framework into understanding the construct of executive functioning. His model postulates that executive functions can be separated into four discrete domains - namely attentional control, information processing, cognitive flexibility and goal setting. In keeping with similar notions on executive functioning, P. Anderson (2002) acknowledges that these domains though discrete, operate in an integrated manner and influence each other. The model is presented diagrammatically below (Figure 1).

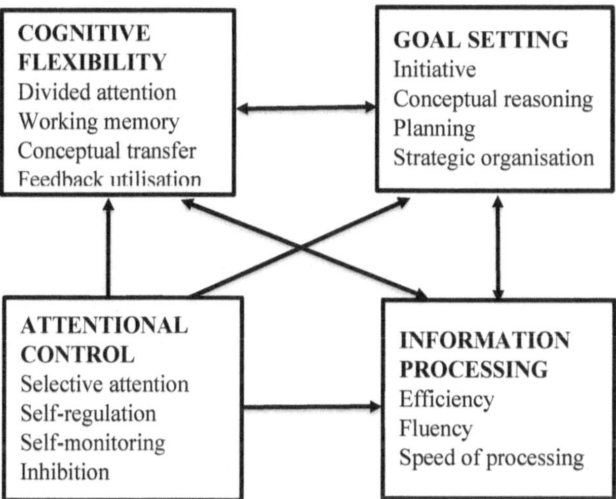

Figure 1. P. Anderson (2002) executive function model

Domain 1: Attentional control. Attentional control encompasses the ability to selectively direct one's attention to specific information in spite of competing stimuli and distractions. This domain encapsulates one's ability to inhibit automatized or instinctual responses. Attentional control further represents the ability to sustain one's attention for an extended period of time, as well as the ability to regulate and monitor responses necessary for the execution of plans (P. Anderson, 2002). It follows, then, that attentional control is critical in adhering to procedure, error monitoring, and achievement of goals. It is also not surprising that individuals with attentional control impairments may exhibit lack of self-control, be impulsive, make mistakes and fail to correct them and leave tasks unfinished (P. Anderson, 2002).

Domain 2: Information processing. Information processing comprises fluency, efficiency and promptness at which input information is produced (P. Anderson, 2002). Fluent output in this regard is denoted by efficiency in which speech is generated. In general, information processing integrity is judged by the promptness, volume and quality of the information released.

Domain 3: Cognitive flexibility. Cognitive flexibility encompasses the ability to switch between different tasks and activities and adapt behaviour and responses to changing stimuli and changes in rules (P. Anderson, 2002). A key component of cognitive flexibility is working memory which denotes the ability to consciously process information in short term memory (P. Anderson, 2002; Diamond, 2013). Cognitive flexibility further encompasses feedback utilisation which refers to the ability to evaluate and gain insight from mistakes; and conceptual transfer which refers to the ability to reconceptualise and formulate new strategies, attend and process different portals of information simultaneously (P. Anderson, 2002).

Domain 4: Goal setting. Goal setting is defined as the ability to be creative and generate new concepts and strategies, and plan the steps necessary to execute these strategies in an efficient and organized manner (P. Anderson, 2002). A key component of goal setting is planning which underlies many aspects of everyday living. Planning encompasses the capacity to select choices among alternatives, organize and appropriately sequence behaviour towards accomplishing a specific goal (Cattie et al., 2012). Another feature of the goal setting domain is conceptual reasoning which speaks to the capacity to abstract central themes from stimuli that may be presented as outwardly discrete and unrelated (P. Anderson, 2002).

Executive dysfunction associated with HIV. Given that executive functioning underlies much of everyday living, impairment in this domain is associated with significant deficits (Diamond, 2013). I also use P. Anderson's (2002) executive function model to discuss some of the prominent deficits associated with an HIV diagnosis.

Attentional control. Research shows that an HIV diagnosis often produces difficulties in attentional control (Nichols et al., 2016). For example, a study by Koekkoek et al. (2008) of 22 adolescents aged between 6 and 17 who had contracted HIV perinatally reported that the HIV-positive adolescents performed poorly on a task that assessed attentional control, relative to controls. This study found that the HIV-positive adolescents were not only slower than the controls, but that they made more errors than what was considered age appropriate, which may reflect poor error monitoring. Poor error monitoring is commonly associated with poor attentional control (P. Anderson, 2002).

Information processing speed. Information processing deficits generally depict a slowness that pervades mental output. This slowness is usually clinically illustrated by hesitancy of output and overall reduction in output production (P. Anderson, 2002). A study by Koekkoek et al. (2008) of a sample of HIV-positive adolescents observed markedly reduced information processing speed in the performance of the adolescents. Similar findings were reported by Nagarajan et al. (2012), with significantly poorer processing speed reported for the sample of 16 HIV-positive adolescents than for the 14 matched HIV-negative controls. Likewise, a South African study found information processing deficits in a sample of HIV-positive adolescents (n = 30) when contrasted with an HIV-negative matched sample of adolescents (n = 69). Consistent with previous research, the study attributed its finding to HIV's predilection for the frontostriatal circuitry, which plays a significant role in the ability to process information (Fraser, 2014).

Cognitive Flexibility. HIV- related deficits in cognitive flexibility include failure to adapt to new expectations, being rigid and inflexible in thought, preferring rituals and procedure because of an inability to adapt to change. Individuals who are impaired in this domain commonly engage in perseverative conduct and tend to repeat mistakes (P. Anderson, 2002). For example a study by Cohen et al. (2015) on a sample of HIV-positive adolescents (n = 35) (between 8 and 18 years) with healthy controls (n = 37) matched for age, sex and SES found that the HIV-positive adolescents struggled with cognitive flexibility mainly due to poorer working memory when compared to their healthy controls (n = 37).

Furthermore, a study by Nichols et al. (2016) reported that adolescents (between 9 and 19 years) who had contracted HIV prenatally, performed more poorly on a switching task, relative to controls, which may be indicative of difficulties with shifting between tasks, which is a component of cognitive flexibility (P. Anderson, 2002). The controls in this study were, however, adolescents that were prenatally exposed to HIV, but uninfected, which literature notes are not ideal controls as they too present with cognitive deficits (Jankiewicz et al., 2017; Nichols et al., 2016).

Goal setting. Impairment in this domain commonly presents in the form of poor problem solving and planning, poor reasoning, disorganised behaviour and a dependence on previous strategies despite an awareness of risks associated with them (P. Anderson, 2002). Fujiwara, Tomlinson, Purdon, Gill, and Power (2015) report on impairment in decision making of HIV-positive individuals (n = 20) compared to matched HIV-negative controls (n = 20). The study results showed that the HIV-positive individuals exhibited reduced planning and were more likely to make poorer decisions despite the associated risk being explicit. This finding was attributed to impairment in the ability to plan ahead and a reduced ability to pre-empt risk. Although the study was focused on adults, the findings are informative given that adolescents are widely documented in literature to be impulsive and inclined to engage in risky behaviour even outside the context of an HIV diagnosis (Laughton et al., 2013).

Executive functions and socioeconomic status (SES). Besides the neuropathological effects of HIV and resultant neuropsychological sequelae, given that people living with HIV are overrepresented in low SES communities, such environmental effects also need to be considered, especially with outcome domains like executive functions, which are so closely tied to everyday behaviour (Hackman et al., 2015; Noble et al., 2015). Evidence from literature suggests that adolescents present differently, cognitively, depending on their socioeconomic backgrounds (Hackman, Gallop, Evans, & Farah, 2015; Noble et al., 2015). Generally, low SES is associated with poor executive functioning particularly in the domains of working memory, attentional control, inhibition, mental flexibility and planning (Hackman et al., 2015). Additional evidence from brain scans reveal brain structural differences according to SES (Noble et al., 2015). These structural differences appear in diffuse brain regions including frontal, cingulate and temporal cortices in which language and executive functions were noted to be negatively affected (Noble et al., 2015). Hence, individuals with HIV may experience a double hazard, in terms of the direct effects of HIV together with possible environmental effects (Hackman et al., 2015; Noble et al., 2015; Lawson & Farah, 2017).

Adolescence

Adolescence, which according to WHO is the developmental stage from age 10 – 19 (WHO, 2018), is widely regarded as the period where significant growth and refinement of executive functioning occurs (Dumontheil, 2015; Laughton et al., 2013; Romer, Reyna, & Satterthwaite, 2017). Affect regulation, which is also a component of executive function, is also noted to improve significantly during this stage (Romer, Reyna, & Satterthwaite, 2017). The changes in cognition and affect that occur in adolescence are sub-served by structural changes particularly in the forebrain and temporal cortices which result in marked improvements in mental abilities (Steinberg, 2005).

Adolescent behavioural instability. Despite a general marked improvement in mental abilities at adolescence, there is also evidence of impulsivity and increased HIV risky behaviour during this stage (Romer et al., 2017). This is because adolescents by and large find novel experiences enticing. The attraction to novelty pervades many aspects of adolescent life and contributes to behavioural experimentation and general taking of risks

(Cattie et al., 2012; Reisner et al., 2009; Romer et al., 2017). In the context of HIV, adolescent risky behaviours commonly include unprotected sex and substance abuse, which add to the risk of contracting HIV (Cattie et al., 2012; Nichols et al., 2015; Smith & Wilkins, 2015; Steinberg, 2005). Literature explains that adolescent behaviour is mostly driven by the expectation of a reward, which suggests that adolescents are likely to engage in risky behaviour even while aware of the negative consequences associated with that particular behaviour (Dumontheil, 2015). Romer et al. (2017) adds that adolescents are sensation seekers mainly due to heightened dopaminergic activation at this developmental stage. So compelling is the pull towards sensation fulfilment that adolescents tend to disregard caution and frequently engage in risky behaviour.

Brain development in adolescence. During adolescence the brain undergoes significant brain maturation mainly through the processes of myelination and pruning which is associated with growth and refinement of cognitive ability (Laughton et al., 2013). During adolescence these brain maturation processes are especially pronounced in the prefrontal cortex which is the brain region that is widely regarded as the executive centre for cognition (Romer et al., 2017; Steinberg, 2005).

Myelination is a process that is carried out by oligodendrocytes which produce myelin, a sheath that covers axons and is responsible for regulating axonal transmission by especially ensuring rapid transmission. Myelination of frontal regions commences soon after birth and spans into adolescence and young adulthood and is generally associated with the maturation of key cognitive functions such as processing speed and problem solving (V. A. Anderson et al., 2001; Laughton et al., 2013; Zillmer, Spiers, & Culbertson, 2008).

Pruning essentially refers to the elimination of mostly weak and generally redundant neurons and poorly connected synaptic connections which leads to a more sculpted brain and thus increased efficiency in neuronal connectivity (Romer et al., 2017). Pruning is thought to reach maximal level at adolescence and to occur much more preferentially in the pre-frontal brain region resulting in grey matter decline in this brain region (Romer et al., 2917). It is widely postulated in literature that pruning of neurons at adolescence is largely experience driven which means that it is significantly influenced by experiences that adolescents encounter at this stage. Pruning, like myelination is associated with an improvement in cognitive functions such as abstraction and improved decision making (Noble et al., 2015; Zillmer et al., 2008).

HIV Treatment

The introduction of Highly Active Antiretroviral Therapy (HAART) substantially changed the trajectory and outcomes of HIV by markedly reducing morbidity and mortality rates related to the virus (Giacomet et al., 2003; Heaton et al., 2011; Nachega, Mills, & Schechter, 2010; Spies, Ahmed-Leitao, Fennema-Notestine, Cherner, & Seedat, 2016; Willen, Cuadra, Arheart, Post, & Govind, 2017; Williams et al., 2006). HAART constitutes the prescription of a combination of drugs from at least two drug categories (for example, nonnucleoside reverse transcriptase inhibitors (NNRTI), integrase inhibitors, protease inhibitors (PI)) in the treatment of HIV (Koekkoek, de Sonneville, Wolfs, Licht, & Geelen, 2008; Smith & Wilkins, 2015; Tan & McArthur, 2012). Earlier trials of treatment for children and adolescents used a mono-therapeutic ARV approach, which produced significant clinical improvements noted in both neurologic and neurodevelopmental domains (Chiriboga et al., 2005). However, the use of single-drug therapies eventually had to be scaled down after the onset of drug-resistant HIV strains. These drug-resistant HIV strains severely weakened treatment impact and necessitated a review of treatment protocols (Chiriboga et al., 2005, Smith & Wilkins, 2015). The introduction of combination therapy thus arose from the need to find an efficacious treatment protocol adequately potent to restrain the mutation of drug-resistant HIV strains (Chiriboga et al., 2005). The distinguishing feature of combination therapy is that, unlike single therapies, this mode of treatment attacks the virus at different points of the replication cycle. For this reason, combination drug therapy has significantly reduced disease progression and HIV-related deaths in children and adolescents (Chiriboga et al., 2005; Smith & Wilkins, 2015).

Currently, HAART is the primary treatment approach to HIV infection in adults, adolescents and children. HAART significantly reduces viral replication, improves the integrity of the immune system, and prevents mutations of drug-resistant strains (Chiriboga et al., 2005, Smith & Wilkins, 2015). HAART has also markedly reduced AIDS-related deaths in children and adolescents – with a reported 70% reduction in HIV-positive children since its roll-out (Chesney, 2000; Chiriboga et al., 2005; Mitchell, 2006; Rivera, Frye, Steele, 2014). Another widely recognised benefit of HAART is its remarkable success rate in reducing opportunistic infections, which were the main cause for high mortality rates among children pre-HAART (Rivera et al., 2014). Since combination therapy not only reduces mortality and morbidity in children and adolescents but also helps to preserve the immune system, it has been credited with the maintenance of age appropriate physical growth and neurocognitive development for HIV-positive children and adolescents (Rivera et al., 2014; Smith & Wilkins, 2015).

Adherence to ART.To maintain the positive health outcomes arising from ART, adherence rates of 90-95% are recommended (Hudelson & Cluver, 2015; Nachega et al., 2014; Peltzer & Pengpid, 2013; Reisner et al., 2009). High adherence is considered to be a reliable predictor for viral suppression, slowed disease progression and overall increase in life expectancy (Nachega et al., 2010; Saberi, Mayer, Vittinghoff, & Naar-King, 2014). Conversely, poor adherence rates are linked to increased viral loads and mutations of drug-resistant HIV strains which can ultimately result in treatment failure (Hudelson & Cluver, 2015; Malee et al., 2009; Nachega et al., 2004; Nichols et al., 2016; Waldrop-Valverde et al., 2010). Poor adherence rates may also increase the likelihood of transmission from an unsuppressed viral load (Kim et al., 2014). Unfortunately, poor adherence patterns persist, particularly among adolescents and threaten to unravel the vast benefits of ART (Kim et al., 2014; Laughton et al., 2013; Nichols et al., 2016).

Factors that impact on adolescent adherence to ART. Literature cites different factors for poor adherence among adolescents. These consist of physical factors which include HIV-related motor disability and side effects from ART which often deter optimal adherence (Malee et al., 2008; Nichols et al., 2012; Smith & Wilkins, 2015). Psychosocial factors such as stigma are additionally noted to impact negatively on adherence patterns among adolescents; notably, psychosocial and physical factors often intersect (Chan et al., 2015; Simbayi et al., 2007; Williams, 2014). However, of these factors, cognitive factors, specifically executive dysfunction, appears to be often implicated as a key contributing factor to adolescents' poor adherence patterns.

Executive dysfunction and adherence. An inverse relationship between adherence to ART and executive dysfunction is often portrayed in literature; where greater executive function impairment is associated with poorer adherence to ART (Waldrop-Valverde, Jones, Gould, Kumar, & Ownby, 2010). This is because executive functions are essential in managing often rigorous medical treatment plans and in keeping up with regular appointments to health facilities (Cattie et al., 2012; Nichols et al., 2016; Waldrop-Valverde et al., 2010). Specifically, literature suggests that adolescents with HIV tend to struggle with processing information related to their medication and also with planning for their medication due to executive dysfunction (Fraser, 2014; Laughton et al., 2015; Nichols et al., 2016). Deficits in processing speed negatively impact adherence to ART in two main ways. First, when processing speed is compromised the ability to adequately process and understand complex medication stipulations becomes compromised (Barclay et al., 2010; Laughton et al., 2015; Nichols et al., 2016). Secondly, when mental processes are slowed, difficulties in absorbing new information such as dosage changes, which are common in ART, may present thus affecting adherence negatively (Barclay et al., 2010; Laughton et al., 2015; Nichols et al., 2016). Another prominent executive dysfunction characteristic that HIV-positive adolescents are often faced with is difficulties in goal setting especially planning. Establishing goals and planning the required steps to meet these goals is often an area HIV-positive adolescents struggle with. Planning difficulties in HIV-positive adolescents often present as a failure to efficiently incorporate medication uptake into their daily schedules. Invariably, these planning difficulties are thought to manifest as lowered adherence patterns (Cattie et al., 2012; Laughton et al., 2015; Nichols et al., 2016).

Measurement of Adherence. Diverse methods of measuring adherence are reported in literature and these broadly fall into three categories (Reisner et al., 2009).

Subjective measurement method. This type of measurement includes the use of self-reports, collateral reports from others e.g., caregivers. Although this method is widely used in research on ART adherence patterns, its major drawback is that it is highly reliant on cognitive competency, which is often compromised in HIV-positive individuals; and also, this method is susceptible to social desirability bias (Gaifer & Boulassel; Reisner et al., 2009). However, this method is useful when exploring or investigating barriers to non-adherence (Gaifer & Boulassel, 2019).

Pharmacologic measurement method. This type of measurement includes pill count, medical records of refills and the use of computerised monitoring systems of pill usage e.g., insertion of microchips in pill containers (Gaifer & Boulassel, 2019). A key advantage of this method is that its effectiveness is not dependent on the cognitive abilities of patients which may eliminate a degree of subjectivity. This method is also a useful predictor for HIV virologic failure in that with this method it is easier to determine if a rise in viral load stems from poor compliance patterns or ART failure (Gaifer & Boulassel, 2019).

Physiological measurement method. This method includes measurements of plasma viral load levels, CD4+ count and ancillary laboratory analysis reports (Hermetet-Lindsay, 2017). Viral load as a marker for adherence has been used widely in research, the outcomes of which suggest that it is a good indicator of the efficacy of ART (Hermetet-Lindsay, 2017, Margot et al., 2018, Nichols et al., 2016; Shoko & Chikobvu, 2019). This method is also considered useful in determining disease progression and in predicting clinical outcomes

(Shoko & Chikobvu, 2019). However, the standard threshold at which viral load suppression is achieved, which would suggest good adherence, varies according to the assays or laboratories used to assess plasma specimens. Generally, though, undetectable plasma readings of viral load are those ≤ 20 copies/ml or in some cases ≤ 50 copies/ml (Hermetet-Lindsay, 2017, Margot et al., 2018, Shoko & Chikobvu, 2019; Williams, 2006). Despite its advantages, this method is however costly (Shoko & Chikobvu, 2019).

Summary and Conclusion

HIV typically enters the brain soon after infection and once in the brain HIV replicates itself resulting in a weakened immune system (Smith & Wilkins, 2015; WHO, 2019). However, overtime, major milestones have been achieved in relation to treating and managing HIV infection such that HIV is now considered a manageable chronic disease (WHO, 2019). Of these milestones, the introduction of ART has had a major impact on efforts aimed towards combatting HIV/AIDS through mainly reducing HIV-related morbidity and mortality rates (UNAIDS, 2018; WHO, 2019). Adherence is however key in gaining maximum impact of ART. Besides physical and psychosocial challenges, frequently reported in the literature, emerging literature also seems to suggest that executive dysfunction may undermine optimal adherence to ART.

Despite adolescents being at a heightened risk for HIV infection and exhibiting marked deficits in HIV-related executive function as well as higher rates of non-adherence, there is a general dearth of research that focusses on this population (Laughton et al., 2013). Moreover, there is even less attention given in research on potential associations between executive functioning and adherence patterns within this population specifically. Frequently, research on executive functions in the context of HIV tends to focus on adults (Laughton et al., 2013; Waldrop-Valverde et al., 2010). The tendency to review mainly adult data on executive function provides a limited characterisation of HIV- related executive function across developmental stages mainly because HIV-positive adults and adolescents are at different stages of brain development and therefore adolescents are likely to present uniquely (Hinkin et al., 2004).

Furthermore, existing literature that has explored HIV-related executive dysfunction has tended to measure single domains of this broad neuropsychological construct (e.g., working memory, problem solving) (Phillips et al., 2016). The limitation in relying on a single domain is that it does not effectively capture the broad nature of executive function. Viewing executive function through the lens of a multi-domain or composite approach as the current study has done allows for a more nuanced analysis which can provide better insight into HIV-related executive dysfunction in adolescents (Phillips et al., 2018). Such a comprehensive insight into the profile of executive function deficits in the context of HIV as offered by this study can be helpful for future interventions. Additionally, despite the high rates of non-adherence observed in adolescents generally, to my knowledge, there is no research that has focussed on determining possible correlation between the domains of executive function according to P. Anderson's (2002) executive function model and adherence.

The current study therefore presents a more nuanced executive function composite approach to assessing executive function and adherence in HIV-positive adolescents and matched HIV-negative controls for a better understanding of the impact of HIV on executive functions in adolescents and the possible association with adherence.

Aims and Hypothesis

The aim of this study was to compare the executive function profile of a group of HIV-positive adolescents with that of a matched HIV-negative control group. Using P. Anderson's (2002) model of executive function, executive functions were considered along the four subdomains: attentional control, processing speed, cognitive flexibility and goal setting.

A second aim of the study was to investigate the relationship between executive function and levels of adherence to ART amongst the HIV-positive individuals in the sample.

Hypotheses. The first study hypothesis was that the sample of HIV-positive adolescents would perform more poorly on executive function tests relative to the HIV-negative control adolescents. A second hypothesis was that for the HIV-positive group, higher adherence would be correlated with higher scores on measures of executive functioning.

Methods

Research Design and Setting

The current study was part of a larger study run by the Desmond Tutu HIV Foundation, HlangananiPlus Health Care Transition (HCT) whose main goal was to support HIV-positive adolescents to transition successfully to adult health care.

The current study is a quantitative, cross sectional, between-groups study, with two groups (Field, 2009). The first group includes a sample of HIV-positive adolescents while the second group was a community recruited matched HIV-negative control group. Data collection for the study was carried out at the Hannan Crusaid Clinic at Gugulethu for the HIV-positive group and at the University of Cape Town (UCT) for the control group.

Participants

Recruitment. Participants for the HIV-positive group were recruited from the HlangananiPlus HCT study sample, while participants in the control group were recruited from communities surrounding or in close proximity to, Gugulethu (e.g., Khayelitsha, Nyanga). The recruitment of control participants was through word of mouth, personal contacts, UCT staff members, and some of the participants were asked whether they had friends and relatives who met the study criteria, and if so, to ask such friends or relatives whether they were interested in participating in the study.

Sample. There were 44 participants ($n = 22$ per group) in the study sample aged 14 - 16 years. All participants were isiXhosa first language speakers and were from a low SES background. To ensure homogeneity within the sample, the control participants were matched to the HIV-positive participants on age, home language and SES.

Inclusion criteria. Participants had to meet specific requirements for inclusion into each group.

HIV- positive group. Participants in the HIV-positive group had to be part of the HlangananiPlus HCT project run by the Desmond Tutu HIV Foundation. The HIV diagnoses of these participants had to be determined by a health practitioner. Related to this, participants in the HIV- positive group were to receive both general medical care and their HIV medication from the Hannan Crusaid clinic in Gugulethu.

Control group. The control group included HIV-negative adolescents that had no reported developmental delays or neurological diagnoses that would compromise their CNS performance.

Exclusion criteria. There were specific exclusion criteria for each group.

HIV-positive group. Participants in the HIV-positive group were excluded if they were taking secondary HIV co-morbid medication such as medication for TB or meningitis. The basis for excluding these participants is that taking these medications may compromise adherence to ART because of risk of interaction between the medications and ART (Onyebujoh, Ribeiro & Whalen, 2007). Collateral information acquired by the Desmond Tutu study team from the medical files of participants was used to determine whether there were prescriptions for HIV co-morbid medication.

Additionally, participants who were prenatally exposed to substance use (drugs and alcohol) were excluded. The reason for this exclusion criterion is that a diagnosis or condition that is associated with drug or alcohol usage during pregnancy such as Foetal Alcohol Spectrum Disorder (FASD) may confound existing HIV-related impairment. Generally, prenatal exposure to these substances is linked to developmental delays and CNS impairment (Mattson, Crocker, & Nguyen, 2011). Since the HIV-positive sample was drawn from the HlangananiPlus HCT larger study, this exclusion criteria was mainly determined through self-report in the larger study during recruitment. Parents were asked about their pregnancy with specific probing around whether their children were exposed to alcohol or drugs prenatally.

Control group. The main exclusion criterion for the control group was an HIV diagnosis. To ensure that this study criterion was upheld; a Paediatric Neuropsychology Developmental Questionnaire short form version was completed by all the parents or caregivers of the control participants (See appendix A). In instances where it was not possible to physically distribute the questionnaire to parents and caregivers, the questionnaire was administered telephonically to determine eligibility.

A second criterion was prenatal exposure to substance use (drugs or alcohol). As previously mentioned, exposure to these substances is commonly associated with developmental delays and CNS impairment (Mattson, Crocker, & Nguyen, 2011).

Measures and Apparatus

A demographic questionnaire was distributed for parents and caregivers to assess the SES of participants. However due to poor return of the questionnaire, the assessment measure of SES was replaced with school quintile.

A battery of neuropsychological tests was administered to assess different domains of executive function. These measures included subtests from the Wechsler Abbreviated Scale of Intelligence (Wechsler, 1999); Wechsler Intelligence Scale for children (WISC IV)

(Wechsler, 2004); The Children's Memory Scale (Cohen, 1997); Children's Colour Trails Test (Llorente et al., 2009); Delis Kaplan Executive Function (Delis, Kaplan & Kramer, 2001); NEPSY II (Korkman, Kirk & Kemp, 2007). A full description of these measures is provided next. I also indicate which tests correspond to the executive function domains included in P. Anderson's (2002) model in Table 1 below.

Table 1

Anderson's executive function model

Domain	Tests	Cognitive construct
Cognitive Flexibility:	Numbers backwards (CMS)	Working memory
	Switching (NEPSY-II)	Switching ability
	Verbal fluency condition 3 (DKEFS)	Switching ability
	Verbal fluency switching accuracy (DKEFS)	Switching ability
	Children's colour trails test 2 (CCTT)	Switching ability
Goal Setting:	Towers (DKEFS)	Planning & problem solving
	Similarities (WASI)	Conceptual reasoning (Verbal)
	Matrix reasoning (WASI)	Conceptual reasoning (Visual)
Information Processing:	Coding (WISC)	Processing speed
	Symbol search (WISC)	Processing speed
	Verbal Fluency condition 1&2 (DKEFS)	Verbal fluency
Attentional Control:	Inhibition (NEPSY-II)	Inhibitory control
	Inhibition errors (NEPSY-II)	Self-monitoring/Inhibitory control

Note. Domains taken from P. Anderson (2002) model for executive function

Wechsler Abbreviated Scale of Intelligence (WASI). The WASI was used to assess general intellectual functioning. The WASI was developed to assess general intellectual functioning in individuals from ages 6 to 89, and has four subtests: Vocabulary, Similarities, Block design and Matrix reasoning. All 4 subtests were utilised to obtain the Full Scale Intelligence Quotient (FSIQ). I also calculated the verbal IQ (VIQ) for each participant which is a measurement of both Vocabulary and Similarities; I also obtained a performance IQ

(PIQ) which is a measurement of both Block design and Matrix reasoning. Given the association between intellectual ability and executive function (Brydges, Reid, Fox, & Anderson, 2012), the measurement of IQ was undertaken to exclude and control for the possibility of delays in general intellectual functioning.

The *Vocabulary* subtest has 42-items and it is used to assess language development and vocabulary acquisition. For the initial four items, participants are required to give the names of pictures presented to them. For the rest of the items, the examiner reads out aloud words to individuals for which they are required to provide definitions.

The *Similarities* subtest is a 26-item subtest that assesses verbal concept formation and reasoning. For the initial four items, participants are presented with a page with two rows of pictures. The participant has to identify which picture in the bottom row is thematically related to the pictures in the top row. For the rest of the items, the participant is presented with two words and is required to explain how they are similar.

Block Design is a 13-item subtest that measures perceptual organization, spatial visualization, visual-motor coordination, and the capacity to conceptually perceive the abstract. Participants are presented with three-dimensional cubes with red and white patterns on the sides. They are shown different geometric designs which they are required to replicate using the cubes within a given time.

Matrix reasoning is a 35-item subtest that assesses nonverbal reasoning. In this test participants are required to view and then select a possible missing piece from five options in order to complete a series of incomplete matrices.

Psychometric properties. The content validity of the *WASI* was established when comparing similar items of subtests to corresponding subtests of other Wechsler batteries such as the *WISC-III*. The Vocabulary, Block design and Similarities subtests which are in both the *WASI* and the *WISC-III* demonstrate significant correlations of 0.72, 0.87, and 0.69 respectively. The reliability coefficients between items in the Similarities subtest ranges between 0.81 and 0.91. The FSIQ, PIQ and VIQ correlation coefficients for both batteries are 0.87, 0.76 and 0.82 respectively. Therefore, it can be assumed that the IQ scales and subtests of the WASI and WISC-III measure similar constructs (Wechsler, 1999). Additionally, the *Vocabulary* and *Similarities* subtests as well as the *Matrix Reasoning* subtests all demonstrate significant correlations of between 0.55 and 0.85 and 0.36 to 0.70 respectively.

The WASI has been successfully used in several published studies conducted on South African children and adolescents (Hoare et al., 2016).

Wechsler Intelligence scale for children – Fourth edition (WISC-IV). The WISC-IV is a measure of general intelligence and has been normed and standardized for children and adolescents aged 6 to 16 years. It has ten core and five supplementary subtests and is focussed on testing four main domains, namely, verbal comprehension, perceptual reasoning, working memory and processing speed. For the current study I used the *Coding* and *Symbol Search* subtests to assess processing speed, which forms part of the information processing domain of P. Anderson's (2002) model of executive function.

In the *Coding* subtest participants are expected to copy symbols within numbered geometric boxes (numbered from 1- 9). The participant is expected to draw or insert each symbol corresponding to a specific box number within a given time limit of 120 seconds.

In the *Symbol Search* subtest participants are presented with a target group of two symbols and a search group of five symbols. Participants are asked to indicate whether the target symbols match with any of five symbols in a search group by ticking on either a yes or no box. Participants are given 120 seconds to carry out this task.

Psychometric properties. The internal reliability for the subtests of the WISC-IV ranges from 0.79 to 0.90, while the reliability coefficients of the composite scale ranges between 0.88 and 0.97. The test re-test reliability for the individual subtests ranges from 0.73 to 0.97 and for the composite scales it ranges between 0.86 and 0.93.

The WISC-IV has been successfully used in South African HIV research on paediatric samples (Hoare et al., 2016).

A developmental neurocognitive assessment (NEPSY –II). The NEPSY-II is a battery of 32 subtests designed to assess neurocognitive functionality. The subtests are designed to cover six domains: Language, executive function and attention, visuospatial processing, memory and learning, and social perception. The NEPSY-II has been normed and standardised for children and adolescents aged 5 to 16 years (Korkman, Kirk & Kemp, 2007). I used the *Inhibition and Switching* subtests from the NEPSY-II. The *Inhibition* subtest corresponds with the attentional control domain, while the *Switching* subtest forms part of the cognitive flexibility domain in P. Anderson's (2002) EF model.

The *Inhibition* subtest is used to assess the ability to inhibit automatic responses. The Inhibition test has three conditions or sub-components – Naming, Inhibition and Switching. I used the Inhibition and Switching sub-components for the present study. In the Inhibition condition, participants are asked to give alternate names to the shapes being presented to them. For example, in the stimulus sheet which has squares and circles, participants are expected to respond by saying "circle" when they see a square and to say "square" when they see a circle. The same principle is applied to the directionality of arrows - participants are expected to say the opposite directions for the stimulus sheet showing arrows, for example participants are expected to say "down" for an arrow facing upwards and to say "up" for an arrow facing downwards. Participants are given a time limit of 240 seconds to complete this task. Underlying this ability is attentional control which is one of the domains in P. Anderson's (2002) model for EF.

The *Switching* subtest is used to evaluate an individual's ability to switch between response types. For example, when they are presented with black circles, they are required to name the shape as they see it (e.g., say "circle" or "square" as they see it). However, when they see a white shape regardless of what shape it is, they are required to say the other shape's name (i.e., if it's a white square they are required to respond "circle"). Besides the use of shapes – circles and squares; the same switching principles are applied to arrows (up and down only). When the arrow is black participants are expected to say the correct direction however when it is white they are expected to say the opposite direction. The *Switching* condition has a time limit of 240 seconds. Impairment of this function is suggestive of difficulty with cognitive flexibility which forms part of P. Anderson's (2002) model of EF.

Psychometric properties. The *NEPSY-II* has a strong content and construct validity and established stability across different age groups with stability coefficients that range from 0.62 to 0.89.

The NEPSY has been widely used in South African paediatric research and specifically used as a measure of executive functioning in South African paediatric HIV research (Hoare et al., 2016; Phillips et al., 2016).

Children's Colour Trails Test (CCTT). The CCTT is designed to measure sequencing, flexibility and switching and is normed and standardized for children aged 8 to 16 years (Williams et al., 1995). The CCTT consists of two components (CCTT 1 and CCTT 2). The first component is a sequencing task in which participants are asked to connect numbers by drawing lines between a sequence of numbers distributed around a stimulus sheet (i.e., from 1 to 2, 2 to 3 etc.). Even though both trials were administered, for the current study analyses I only used the findings of the second trial of the CCTT (CCTT 2) whereby participants are presented again with a stimulus sheet with numbers displayed. However, unlike in the first component this time the same number is shown twice on the stimulus sheet in two different colours (yellow and pink). The participant is expected to sequentially join the numbers while alternating the colours (i.e., pink 1 to yellow 2, yellow 2 to pink 3, etc.), and is required to do this task as quickly as possible as completion time is a key indicator of one's ability to switch between responses. The ability to switch between the different colours while keeping to the correct number sequencing is a measurement of cognitive flexibility which is one of the executive function domains outlined in P. Anderson's (2002) model.

Psychometric properties. The reliability and validity of the CCTT 1 and CCTT 2 was examined using a sample of 54 children aged between 6–12-years with ADHD. At 8 and16 week time points results showed a test retest reliability coefficient range of 0.46 - 0.68. To establish factorial validity children with traumatic brain injury (TBI), other types of trauma and healthy controls were assessed. This analysis revealed a 3-factor loading structure; the first factor was categorized as perceptual tracking speed and ease of distractibility, an inability to control impulses and poor attention were identified as Factor 2, and Factor 3, was categorized as difficulty with attention (Llorente et al., 2009).

The CCTT has been used in published studies on South African children and adolescents. In a study by Ferrett et al (2010), researchers used the CCTT as part of their neuropsychological battery to assess the cognitive functioning of adolescents (13-15 years) with an alcohol use disorder. Another South African study on paediatric HIV utilised the CCTT in its cognitive test battery (Hoare et al., 2016).

The Children's Memory Scale (CMS). The CMS includes eight tests designed to primarily measure learning and memory among children aged 5 to 16 years (Cohen, 1997). The Numbers subtest consists of two components: *Numbers Forwards* and *Numbers Backwards*. In *Numbers Forwards* the examiner reads out numbers which participants are expected to repeat back and is used to measure attention. On the other hand, *Numbers Backwards* is used to assess working memory and, in this component, participants are required to repeat the order of numbers as presented by the examiner in reverse order. I only used the *Numbers Backwards* component since working memory is included in the cognitive flexibility domain of P. Anderson's (2002) model of EF.

Psychometric properties. Reliability coefficients for the Numbers subtest range from 0.71 to 0.83. The test re-test reliability for the subtests range from 0.71 to 0.91 and the structure and content validity ranges from 0.06 to 0.96, across all ages. Moreover, the CMS has been found to correlate well with the Wechsler Memory Scale – III (WMS-III), with measurement indices reflecting convergent validity on similar sub-domains.

The CMS has been used with a sample of children aged 8 -18 years for HIV research in USA (Nichols et al., 2012). It has also been used on a South African population for substance abuse research (Ferrett et al., 2010).

Delis-Kaplan Executive Function System (DKEFS). The DKEFS comprises nine subtests and is designed to test executive function in children and adults from age 8 to 89 (Delis, Kaplan & Kramer, 2001). I used two subtests from this test battery: *Verbal fluency* and the *Towers* subtests. Verbal fluency is included in the information processing domain of P. Anderson's (2002) EF model. The *Towers* subtest is used as a measurement of planning and falls under the goal setting domain of the P. Anderson's (2002) EF model. From the Towers subtest I used the achievement score, move accuracy score and the rule violations score.

The *Verbal Fluency* subtest is designed to assess processing speed, verbal retrieval and recall, self-monitoring and inhibition. It consists of three conditions or tasks; a phonemic fluency task (condition 1), semantic fluency task (condition 2), and a switching task (condition 3). In the phonemic fluency task participants are required to generate words beginning with a specified letter. Conventionally, participants are given the letters F, A, and S as the starting letters of the words that they need to generate. I used M, A, and T in this study based on previous local research (Baufeldt, 2009).

In the semantic fluency task participants are expected to generate words within a specified category (animals and the names of boys or girls). Lastly in the switching task participants are required to switch between stimuli (furniture and fruits).

The *Towers* subtest is used to measure goal setting ability, including problem solving, planning abilities and strategic thinking. The test stimuli consists of a board with pegs and 5 discs. The examiner places the discs on the pegs according to the stimulus book item being administered and then invites the participant to arrange the discs on the pegs according to the end arrangement shown in the stimulus book. The participant is expected to reproduce the arrangement as quickly as possible in the fewest number of moves while at the same time adhering to two rules. First, only one of the discs can be moved at a time and second, larger discs may not be placed on top of smaller ones. As the test continues each arrangement increases in complexity and the time given to complete an arrangement increases in length ranging from 30 seconds to 4 minutes.

Psychometric properties. Test-retest coefficients are in the moderate range with great variability among the subtests. Internal consistency, test-retest reliability and validity have been established for each of the DKEFS subtests (Delis et al., 2001).

The DKEFS test battery has been administered on a USA sample of adolescents aged between 9 -19 years comprising of prenatally infected HIV-positive and prenatally HIV exposed but uninfected adolescents (Nichols et al., 2016). The DKEFS Tower test has also been used in South African paediatric HIV research (see Hammond, Eley, Ing, Wilmshurst, 2019).

Paediatric Neuropsychology Developmental Questionnaire (short form version) (PNDQ). This is a screening questionnaire aimed at obtaining information related to participants' developmental history. It incorporates questions that relate to pregnancy and birth to establish whether any complications were experienced at any of these stages. Other questions relate to schooling, to assess if there was any repeating of grades and the reasons, should this have occurred. There are also questions regarding the mental and medical health of participants aimed at establishing whether participants have been referred for mental and medical health reasons and also whether they were on any chronic medication. This questionnaire is a short form of the one used at the local paediatric neuropsychology clinic at the Red Cross War Memorial Children's hospital.

School quintile. The current study used school quintile as a proxy measurement index of SES and quality of education. School quintile is a South African classification for schools and the communities they are located in: 1 being the poorest schools and 5 the wealthiest schools. This classification is based on the type of community in which the school is located; therefore, schools that are classified in low quintiles are commonly subsidised schools in poor communities (Department of Basic Education, 2018).

Viral load. I used plasma HIV viral load as a proxy for adherence, which is a method commonly reported in the literature (Collier et al., 2018; Margot et al., 2018; Shoko & Chikobvu, 2019). Participants' viral load readings were extracted from participants' medical folders at Hannan Crusaid clinic in Gugulethu.

Procedure

Consenting and Assenting. Given that this study formed part of the HlangananiPlus HCT larger study, participants in the HIV-positive group were consented by the HlangananiPlus HCT study team. As part of consenting to participate in the larger study participants were also informed of the aim, procedure, risks and benefits of the current study by either myself or a researcher in the study team of the larger study. The study team of the larger study also presented the participants in the HIV- positive group with consent forms for their parents and caregivers to consider and sign, and the participants themselves were given assent forms before assessments began (see Appendices B and C).

Control participants' parents and caregivers were also given consent forms to consider and sign and, as with the HIV-positive group, the participants themselves were given assent forms to sign (see Appendices D and E). Before signing the consent/assent forms, the study aims, procedure, risks and benefits were explained to both participants and their parents or caregivers. Explanation of the study was carried out in person and telephonically and in all instances an isiXhosa translator was there to assist.

All consent, assent and testing record forms were translated into isiXhosa by the University of Stellenbosch Language Centre; the Language Centre also performed back translation on all the forms to ensure validity and authenticity of translation.

Testing of participants. Testing of the HIV-positive group was carried out at the Hannan Crusaid Clinic in Gugulethu on Friday afternoons and Saturday mornings in an enclosed room to ensure confidentiality. Control participants were tested on Saturdays in the Psychology department at UCT in quiet rooms to ensure confidentiality.

I tested participants together with a two other neuropsychology Masters students and a Psychology Honours student, who assisted. At each testing session there was an interpreter present (see Appendix N for interpreters' details), who was experienced in the administration of the neurocognitive tests, to assist with translation as participants were isiXhosa first language speakers. However, some participants (in both groups) were also fluent in English and despite the presence of an interpreter who translated all instructions in isiXhosa, elected to give their responses in English for some of the neurocognitive tests.

Each testing session lasted for approximately 2 to 2.5 hours per participant including breaks during which participants were provided with refreshments. At the end of testing the control participants received R50 for transport and a R50 food voucher as compensation for their time. Participants in the HIV-positive group were provided with R30 for transport. The transport compensation money for the HIV-positive group was decided as part of the larger HlangananiPlus HCT project on account of the testing site being located within the participants' community. The order of the tests is included in appendix F.

Data Analysis

Data was analysed using SPSS Version 25. Where assumptions underlying statistical tests were violated, the appropriate non-parametric tests were used. For the statistical analysis, the independent variable was the group variable and the dependent (outcome) variables were the executive function scores for the various executive function measures previously described.

For the between-subjects analyses, the executive function scores of the HIV-positive group were compared to that of the control group. I also ran a within-groups analysis based on age at initiation of ART for the group with HIV.

Scoring of neurocognitive data. I scored all the data according to the procedures of the test manuals of each test. I converted all the neuropsychological test variables into age appropriate scaled scores; the only exception was for the CCTT2 score which I left as a raw score measurement of time.

Scaled scores are statistically adjusted raw scores based on the normative performance standards of different tests. Notably, scaled scores are helpful in ascertaining comparability or differences in group performance. Additionally, scaled scores allow for maintenance of consistency in score interpretation particularly when different tests have been utilised (Tan & Michelle, 2011).

Main Analysis. Between-group differences on continuous demographic variables were mainly evaluated using independent samples *t*-tests. In the case of the within group analysis for the HIV-positive group, based on age at initiation of ART, I used a Kruskal-Wallis *H* test, given the group sizes. Chi-square or Fisher's Exact tests (when >20% of expected cell counts are <5) were used to examine categorical variables. Descriptive statistics were computed on the demographics for all participants; this included descriptors such as sex, age, language, school quintile and intellectual ability.

Executive function (EF).

Deriving and comparing composite scores. Due to the large number of dependent variables compared to the small sample size, a hybrid method using composite scores was used (see Ferrett et al. 2010). To do this, the executive function neuropsychology test battery was sorted into composite domains (cognitive flexibility, information processing, attentional control, goal setting) based on P. Anderson's (2002) EF model, and theoretical assumptions and established categorizations. Individual neuropsychological test variables were converted to z-scores, which were categorized into composites for the four domains outlined in P. Anderson's (2002) EF model and averaged to yield an overall composite EF z-score (Medina et al., 2007).

I then assessed whether the EF *z*-scores shared enough variance to be considered one overarching factor. Cronbach's Alpha for the 17 EF subtests was 0.713, indicating that the items sufficiently measure one construct (executive functioning). I further calculated Cronbach's alpha for each EF domain: cognitive flexibility, information processing, attentional control and goal setting. Cronbach's alpha for cognitive flexibility was 0.75, for information processing, 0.83, for attentional control, 0.84, and for goal setting, 0.69, indicating that the tests in these domains sufficiently measure the same / similar construct.

Effect size. To measure effect size, I used Cohen's *d.* Small, medium and large effect sizes, are represented by values of 0.2, 0.5, and 0.8 respectively (Field, 2009). This effect size was useful in assessing the magnitude of the results obtained.

Correlations. I was also interested in assessing associations between adherence for the HIV-positive group, measured by viral load, and executive function scores. Therefore, I computed correlations between the four executive function domains and adherence using Pearson's *r*. I grouped the viral load data into three: group 1 were participants with a low detectable viral load and a viral load < 20 copies/ml; group 2 were participants with a viral load > 20 copies/ml but < 2,500 copies/ml, and group 3 were participants who had a viral load > 80,000 copies/ml. The groupings of viral loads were then correlated with the composite executive function scores.

Missing data. Where there was missing data, I excluded the cases pairwise. This means that participants with missing data were excluded, but only for specific analyses (Field, 2009).

Outliers. Individual test scores that scored either above or below the mean by at least two standard deviations were identified as outliers and were excluded from the analyses (Field, 2009). I do include the results both before and after the removal of outliers though in order to promote transparency. Outliers are extreme values that lie far away from the observed distribution pattern of data points. By nature, outliers tend to introduce bias in the computation of test statistics resulting in either overestimated or underestimated statistical values (Kwak & Kim, 2017; Laurikkala et al., 2000).

Ethical Considerations

I received ethical clearance from both the University of Cape Town's Psychology Department Research Ethics Committee and the Faculty of Health Sciences Human Research Ethics Committee (HREC) (see Appendix G & H). Regarding HREC clearance, the current study's ethical provisions were incorporated into the HlangananiPlus HCT larger project's overall ethical protocol. An ethical amendment to include community controls was approved by the University of Cape Town's Psychology Department Research Ethics Committee. The control data was collected as part of an Honours research project by Bryony Dyssell, which was linked to, and a pilot study for, the current study (see Appendix I). I was fully involved in the running of that preliminary (pilot) study.

Consent, voluntary participation and confidentiality. Written consent and assent was obtained from parents/caregivers and participants, respectively. Participants and parents/caregivers were told of the voluntary nature of participating in this study and that there would be no negative repercussions should they opt to withdraw from the study at any point.

Confidentiality and anonymity. Participants were assured of confidentiality and anonymity regarding all data collected. Participants' names during data extraction and analysis were replaced with participant identity numbers (PIDs) to ensure anonymity. Data was treated confidentially and access to study records was limited to myself, my supervisor and co-supervisor, and those directly involved in the research. Study records were further kept in locked cabinets and in computers with password access codes.

Risks, benefits and compensation.

Risks. Participants were not exposed to physical, psychological or social risks in the study. However, due to extended testing sessions some participants may have become fatigued. Where this was observed intermittent breaks with light refreshments were held.

Benefits. The key benefit of the study was the valuable knowledge that was gained from the research regarding the impact of HIV on executive function in HIV-positive adolescents and also the influence of non-neurologic factors on cognitive functioning in healthy controls.

Compensation. Participants in the HIV-positive group received R30 as compensation for transport, given that testing was carried out within their community; they also received refreshments during breaks. Testing of control participants took place outside of their communities, at UCT, therefore they received R50 towards transport as well as a R50 food voucher for refreshments.

Results

Sample characteristics

The HIV-positive participants in the current study sample were all prenatally infected with HIV. Ten (10) of them were initiated on ART before age 5; five (5) started treatment on ARVs between age 6 – 10, and four (4) participants after age 10. The date of treatment inception was not included in the medical files of 3 participants. Although this was not one of the aims of the study, a review of the means for the three groups based on age of initiation of ART, showed no real variance, and a Kruskal-Wallis *H* test, showed no significant within-group variance based on this variable ($p \geq .164$) for age and across all composites.

Descriptive statistics were computed for all the demographic variables for both the HIV-positive and Control groups to determine sample characteristics. These are outlined in Table 1. There were no significant between-group differences for any of the demographic variables (all *p*'s > .150). This result indicates that the sample demographic characteristics have not disproportionately influenced the executive function outcome variables. No statistics were performed for home language since all participants were isiXhosa first language speakers.

Table 1

Sample Demographic Statistics (N = 44)

	HIV group		Control group		Test Statistics		
	n	*M (SD)/ratio*	*n*	*M (SD)/ratio*	t/χ^2	*p*	ESE[a]
Age (months)	22	185.13 (10.82)	22	183.55 (9.58)	-0.52	.609	0.15
Sex (F:M)	22	15:7	22	18:4	1.09	.296	0.16
Quintile[b] (1-5)	21	3.00[c] (0.71)	22	2.68 (0.72)	-1.47	.150	0.45
Fee-paying (Y:N)	21	3:18	22	1:21	[d]	.345	0.17

Note. ESE – Estimate Effect Size. [a]ESE - Cohen's *d* for independent sample *t*-tests and Cramer's *V* for chi-square tests of contingency. [b]Quintile – South African public school ranking system based on the wealth of the surrounding community (1 being the poorest and 5 being the wealthiest) to determine learner subsidisation. Data was retrieved from the Department of Basic Education (DBE, 2018). [c]One HIV participant did not provide name of their school; therefore, the sample size was reduced to $n = 21$. [d]Fisher's Exact Test performed because > 20% of expected cells counts < 5.

General intellectual functioning

As reflected in Table 2, there were no significant between-group differences in terms of general intellectual functioning outcomes for the HIV and Control groups (all *p's* > .148).

The mean scores VIQ, PIQ, and consequently, FSIQ, fall within the borderline range for both groups, however, the means for the HIV-positive group are expectedly lower than that of the control group.

Table 2

General intellectual ability outcomes: between-group comparisons HIV positive group vs controls (N = 44)

	HIV group		Control group		Test Statistics		
	n	*M (SD)*	*n*	*M (SD)*	*t*	*p*	ESE[a]
PIQ	22	75.09 (13.17)	22	78.55 (14.48)	0.83	.206	0.25
VIQ	22	72.59 (11.67)	22	75.45 (12.52)	0.79	.218	0.24
FSIQ	22	71.50 (11.80)	22	75.23 (11.51)	1.06	.148	0.32

Note. Means are presented with standard deviations in parentheses.
[a]ESE is Cohen's *d* (0.2- small, 0.5- medium, 0.8- large). PIQ: Performance intelligence quotient; VIQ: Verbal intelligence quotient; FSIQ: Full scale intelligence quotient.

Executive function composites

The individual subtests that make up each of the four domains (cognitive flexibility, information processing, attentional control and goal setting) are shown in Appendix K.

Before the removal of outliers. Table 3 presents the neuropsychological test performance of the HIV group and Control group before the removal of outliers. There were no significant between-group differences in terms of the individual composite executive function variables (all *p's* > .084). The effect sizes were all small.

Table 3

Executive function composites: between-group comparisons HIV group vs Controls (before removal of outliers)

	HIV group		Control group		Test Statistics		
	n	*M (SD)*	*n*	*M (SD)*	*t*	*p*	ESE[a]
Composite scores							
Cognitive Flexibility[a]	20	-0.05 (0.61)	22	<.001 (0.55)	0.27	.394	0.09
Goal Setting	22	-0.02 (0.63)	22	<.001 (0.61)	0.08	.467	0.03
Information Processing[b]	21	-0.34 (0.76)	22	<.001 (0.82)	1.41	.084	0.43
Attentional Control	22	-0.26 (0.97)	22	<.001 (0.92)	0.93	.180	0.28
EF Total[c]	20	-0.12 (0.47)	22	<.001 (0.53)	0.74	.233	0.24

Note. Means are presented with standard deviations in parentheses. [a]ESE is Cohen's d (0.2- small, .5- medium, 0.8- large). [b]Cognitive flexibility: 2 participants from the HIV group did not complete the switching task included in the composite score for cognitive flexibility. [c]Information processing: 1 participant from the HIV group did not complete the verbal fluency task included in the composite score for information processing. EF – Executive function. [d]EF Total: The EF score could not be computed for 2 participants from the HIV group due to non-completion of tasks.

Removal of outliers. Executive function composite scores > 2SD above or < 2SD below the mean were identified as outliers and were removed (Field, 2009). Thus, four adolescents from the HIV-positive group were removed listwise from the data analysis because they scored > 2 SD above the mean on their executive function test composites (one on cognitive flexibility, one on processing speed, and two on the EF total). One Control adolescent was removed from the data analysis because they scored > 2 SD above the mean on the cognitive flexibility composite.

Table 4 presents the data of the Control and HIV-positive group after removal of the outliers. The results show that adolescents with HIV performed significantly worse on Information Processing ($p = .042$) with a moderate effect size of 0.55. The results further showed a trend for the HIV-positive group to perform worse on the total executive function score ($p = .068$), with a moderate effect size.

Table 4

Executive function composites: between group comparisons HIV group vs controls (after the removal of outliers)

	HIV group		Control group		Test Statistics		
	n	*M (SD)*	*n*	*M (SD)*	*t*	*p*	*ESE*
Composite scores							
Cognitive Flexibility	19	-0.14 (0.49)	21	-0.07 (0.46)	0.46	.325	0.15
Goal Setting	22	-0.02 (0.63)	22	<.001 (0.61)	0.08	.467	0.03
Information Processing	20	-0.42 (0.69)	22	<.001 (0.82)	1.78	.042*	0.55
Attentional Control	22	-0.26 (0.97)	22	<.001 (0.92)	0.93	.180	0.28
EF Total	18	-0.22 (0.36)	22	<.001 (0.53)	1.52	.068	0.48

Note. Means are presented with standard deviations in parentheses. ESE is Cohen's d (0.2- small, 0.5- medium, 0.8- large)

Correlations between executive function composites and adherence

Correlations between adherence and executive function composites were computed for the HIV-positive group. A log function was computed to minimise the effects of the large variance in the viral load data. 61% of the adolescents had low detectable viral load and viral loads of <20 copies/ml. Of the adolescents who had a detectable viral load, 3 participants had extremely high viral loads > 80,000 copies/ml. For the adolescents who had a detectable viral load, the median was 2454 (IQR: 140 – 146091). Viral load was not significantly correlated with any executive function composite variables (all *ps* > .068) (see Table 5). However, Pearson's correlation coefficient for goal setting and viral load is medium. It is also in the expected direction in that a negative association between goal setting and viral load is indicated. An unexpected finding was a positive correlation between attentional control, information processing, total executive function score and viral load. The associated effect sizes were however small.

Table 5

Correlations between Viral Load and Executive Function Composite Scores

	VL	Cognitive Flexibility	Goal Setting	Attentional control	Information Processing	EF Total
VL	1.00	-.135	-.328	.074	.123	.075
p-value		.291	.068	.371	.303	.384

Note. Pearson's correlation co-efficient; Small: 0.1- 0.3; Medium: 0.3 - 0.5; Large: 0.5 - 1

Figure 1, below, is a visual presentation of total executive function scores and viral load. High scores of total executive function are not consistently associated with low viral load (high adherence marker). Participants with high viral loads that exceeded 80,000 copies/ml (group 3.00) attained composite executive function scores that were proportionate to participants with low detectable viral loads and < 20 copies/ml (group 1). Adherent participants (with low viral loads) also scored poorly on executive functioning.

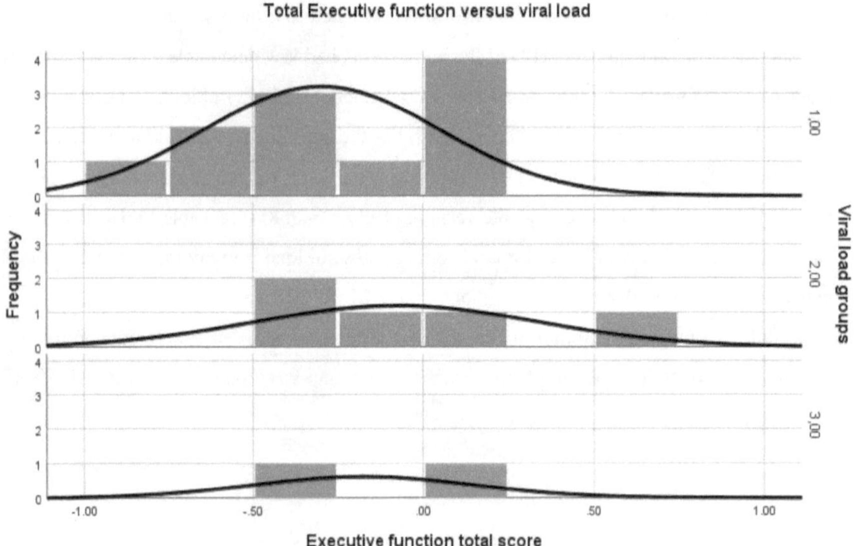

Figure 2. Visual representation of viral data and executive function total scores

Discussion

This study was part of a larger study, HlangananiPlus HCT (see Appendix M for details of study team), run by the Desmond Tutu HIV Foundation. The goal of the HlangananiPlus HCT study was to facilitate the transition of HIV-positive adolescents from youth to adult health care services. This goal came about after the Desmond Tutu HIV Foundation realised that the success rate of transitioning HIV-positive adolescents into adult health care services was poor and led to a rise in markedly poor patterns of adherence once they reached young adulthood (Desmond Tutu HIV Research Foundation, 2017). Poor adherence to ART among HIV-positive individuals is a serious concern, because it risks the vast health benefits gained from the roll out of HIV therapy (Heaton et al., 2011; Hudelson & Cluver, 2015; Inzaule, Hamers, Kityo, Rinke De Wit, & Roura, 2016; Willen, Cuadra, Arheart, Post, & Govind, 2017). These health benefits include a decline in the emergence of HAND as well as a significant decline in the manifestation of opportunistic infections and an overall increase in life expectancy (Nachega, Mills, & Schechter, 2010; Williams et al., 2006; Spies, Ahmed-Leitao, Fennema-Notestine, Cherner, & Seedat, 2016; Heaton et al., 2015; Willen et al., 2017).

Poor adherence to ART, if not addressed, can also typically lead to negative health outcomes that manifest physically and/or cognitively (Heaton et al., 2011). Given HIV's partiality for frontal cortices including frontal circuitries and deep white matter, it is not surprising that the neuropsychological profile associated with HIV infection, would prominently feature executive dysfunction. I used P. Anderson's (2002) executive function model, which divides executive functions into four main domains (attentional control, processing speed, cognitive flexibility and goal setting), as the theoretical framework for this study, to investigate the impact of an HIV diagnosis on executive functioning in adolescents.

The aims of the current study were twofold. The first aim was to investigate between-group differences in executive functioning between HIV-positive adolescents and matched HIV-negative controls. Executive function scores were derived for each of the four domains depicted in P. Anderson's (2002) executive function model for each group and an overall executive function score was computed by averaging the scores of the individual executive function domain scores. The hypothesis for this aim was that the sample of HIV-positive adolescents would perform more poorly on executive function tests relative to the HIV-negative control group. The second aim was to determine whether there were associations between adherence and outcomes on measures of executive function, again with a focus on the domains put forward in P. Anderson's (2002) model. I hypothesized that there would be a negative association between adherence (lower viral load) and executive function performance and that this association would be significant.

Summary of Results

In terms of the results, there were no significant differences in demographics or general intellectual functioning between the study groups. Regarding aim 1, apart from processing speed (after the removal of outliers) there were no significant between-group differences in executive functioning outcomes that emerged between the two study groups. Related to this finding was that the scores of the executive function tests for both groups were lower than the normative scores of the tests, by at least 2SDs below the tests' means. The effect sizes across the executive function domains ranged from small to medium suggestive that the study was underpowered, and this might contribute to the lack of significant between-group differences. There are, however, other possible reasons that one may conjecture to explain these findings and these reasons are elaborated on further on in this discussion.

Regarding aim 2, the correlations between adherence and executive functioning outcomes did not produce any significant associations for each of the executive function composites. However, the correlation coefficients between cognitive flexibility and adherence (viral load), goal setting and adherence were negative and thus in keeping with my hypothesis. Across the executive function domains, the effect sizes ranged from small to medium. Specifically, the effect sizes for cognitive flexibility, attentional control and information processing were small; however, the effect size for goal setting was in the medium range.

General Intellectual Functioning

There were no significant between-group differences in general intellectual functioning for the HIV- positive and Control groups, and the associated effect sizes were small. Although the mean differences of the groups are not significant, the finding of low mean scores for the HIV-positive group, at least descriptively, compared to the Control group, is in accordance with other studies which also found that HIV-positive adolescents perform poorly when compared to controls in general intellectual functioning (Cohen et al., 2015; Hoare et al., 2016; Smith et al., 2012).

An important result that emerged from the outcomes for this domain is that the mean scores of both groups were in the borderline range (see Appendix J for the qualitative descriptions of the WASI results). Here one takes into account the reported discrepancies in performance for individuals from low- to middle-income country contexts when their scores are compared to Western normative data (Shuttleworth-Edwards et al., 2013).

A review of general intellectual ability is important in a study on executive function given that previous research has noted an association between intelligence and executive function. Some lines of research point out that intellectual ability is partially mediated by executive function and that the relationship between intellectual ability and executive function is explained by the constructs both being predominantly sub-served anatomically by the prefrontal cortex (Brydges, Reid, Fox, & Anderson, 2012).

Aim 1: To Compare Executive Functioning Outcomes on Neuropsychological Tests, of HIV-positive Adolescents and HIV-negative Controls

The findings for aim 1 are inconsistent with the outcomes of several other studies which report that HIV-positive adolescents, when compared to HIV-negative controls, perform more poorly on assessments of various executive functions (Nichols et al., 2015b). For example, in their study, Cohen et al. (2016) found that HIV-positive children and adolescents performed significantly more poorly on processing speed, working memory and general intellectual ability outcomes; the authors attributed these findings to HIV-induced reductions in both white and grey matter volume. Additionally, Hoare et al. (2016) also found deficiencies in processing speed and cognitive flexibility among HIV-positive adolescents compared to matched controls. Similarly, Boivin et al. (2018) found that HIV-positive children when compared to their HIV-negative peers performed poorly on problem solving, planning, processing speed and abstraction. Collectively, these studies suggest executive dysfunction in HIV-positive individuals across the subdomains that make up the core components in Anderson's (2002) model.

Attentional control. For the purposes of this study and based on P. Anderson's (2002) EF model, I used measures of inhibition for this domain. Inconsistent with previous literature, this study found no between group differences in this domain with a small effect size. Findings from international studies show that HIV-positive adolescents' performance is compromised in this domain (Koekkoek, de Sonneville, Wolfs, Licht, & Geelen, 2008; Nichols et al., 2015) . For example, the study by Koekkoek et al. (2008) found that Dutch HIV-positive children and adolescents performed significantly lower than Dutch national norms in a test that measured attentional control. Even though the Koekkoek et al. (2008) study did not have controls and only measured performance against national normative scores, it is comparable to the current study with regard to the participants' age range (6 -17 years). A study by Ruel et al. (2012) of 267 Ugandan children (6 – 12 years) also found that

HIV-positive children exhibited difficulties with attention when compared to HIV-negative controls. This finding was attributed to high plasma viral load which was determined by a plasma viral load level that exceeded the median of the study cohort. Even though the age of the participants in the Ruel et al. (2012) study fall outside of the age range of the current study, that study context also being SSA, suggests contextual comparisons with the current study.

Cognitive flexibility. For the purposes of this study and, based on P. Anderson's (2002) EF model, I used measures of working memory and switching for this domain. Contrary to the expectation that there would be between group differences in this domain, this study found none, and the effect size was negligible. According to evidence from international and local studies, HIV-positive adolescents exhibit difficulty on tests that measure mental flexibility (Cohen et al., 2015; Hoare et al., 2016; Nichols et al., 2015). For example, Hoare et al. (2016), using a South African sample found that HIV-positive children and adolescents (aged 6 - 16 years) performed more poorly in a test of cognitive flexibility (CCTT test) than HIV-negative matched controls. Also inconsistent with the current study, the investigation by Cohen et al. (2015) of a Dutch sample found that HIV-positive children and adolescents (8 – 18 years old) performed significantly worse on a working memory test than matched HIV-negative controls. Like the current study, the Cohen et al. (2015) study used the WISC Digit Span subtest to measure working memory and their study design also included healthy controls. Brain scans in Cohen et al.'s (2016) study revealed that the HIV-positive group had smaller brain volumes than the controls evidenced specifically in reduced brain grey matter volumes which correlated with the observed deficits in working memory. Similarly, recent research by Lewis-de los Angeles et al. (2017) of HIV-positive American adolescents (mean age 16.7 years) also reported that HIV-related smaller brain volumes correlated with difficulties in working memory.

Goal setting. For the purposes of this study, and based on Anderson's (2002) model, I used measures of planning and abstraction for this domain. There were no significant between-group differences found in this domain and the effect size was negligible. Contrastingly, some international and local studies have found that HIV-positive adolescents struggle with goal setting and planning (Laughton, Cornell, Boivin, & Van Rie, 2013; Phillips et al., 2016). Goal setting and planning are interdependent components in that goal setting encompasses designing strategies for the attainment of specific outcomes and is directly linked to decision making, and planning involves the ability to identify and conceptualise sequences and integration of behaviour to accomplish a specific goal (Anderson, 2002; Cattie et al., 2012).

Research by Lewis-de los Angeles et al. (2017) of 40 prenatally-infected American adolescents (mean age 16.7 years) and 334 HIV uninfected controls (mean age 16.1 years) reported planning and abstraction difficulties in the HIV group. That study attributed the observed planning and abstraction difficulties to HIV-related cortical thinning in frontal brain regions seen in brain scans of the HIV-positive group. The difficulties with planning and abstraction were noted to contribute to poor decision making and risky behaviour in the HIV group. Impairment in planning and conceptual reasoning has also been reported in a longitudinal study by Boivin et al. (2018), which focussed on children aged (6 – 11 years). This was a multi-site study and included 611 children from South Africa, Malawi, Uganda and Zimbabwe. In this study there were HIV-positive children ($n = 246$), HIV exposed but uninfected ($n = 183$), and HIV unexposed ($n = 182$) children. The findings of that study showed that, of all the groups, the HIV-positive children performed most poorly cognitively, in the domains of planning and reasoning. The study attributed these executive difficulties to stunted growth and wasting as a developmental effect of poverty and HIV as well as to a pervasive late start in ART.

In general, there is a dearth of literature on HIV-related planning deficits specific to adolescents. A large body of literature focuses on adult populations (Cattie et al., 2012; Fujiwara, Tomlinson, Purdon, Gill, & Power, 2015; Waldrop-Valverde, Jones, Gould, Kumar, & Ownby, 2010). HIV-positive

Processing speed. For the purposes of this study, and based on Anderson's (2002) model, I used measures of verbal fluency and processing speed for this domain. Initially, this study found no significant between-group differences in this domain. However, after removing four participants who performed >2SD above the mean on composite EF tests from the sample (and were therefore, in effect, outliers), significant group differences were observed with a moderate effect size. Specifically, results showed that the HIV-positive group had a slower processing speed than the control group. This finding is consistent with a large body of research which has established that HIV-positive adolescents perform poorly in neuropsychological tests of processing speed (Boivin et al., 2018; Cohen et al., 2015; Hoare et al., 2016; Koekkoek et al., 2008). Koekkoek et al. (2008) found that a sample of Dutch HIV perinatally-infected children and adolescents between the ages of 6 – 17 performed below age appropriate Dutch test norms on tests of processing speed. Although this study by Koekkoek et al. (2008) did not have controls, it was comparable to this study in that the age range of the participants of that study encompass the age range of the present study. A study by Cohen et al. (2016) of Dutch and SSA HIV-positive children and adolescents (aged 8 -18) found that the HIV-positive group (*n* = 35) performed significantly poorly when compared to matched healthy controls (*n* = 37) on tests that measured processing speed. The deficit was attributed to HIV-related grey matter atrophy and extensive white matter brain lesions identified on brain scans of the HIV-positive group.

Processing speed is a salient HIV-related CNS feature mainly owing to a direct effect of the impact of the virus on brain white matter (Boivin et al., 2018; Fellows, Byrd, & Morgello, 2014; Koekkoek et al., 2008; Nagarajan et al., 2012; Sarma et al., 2014; Woods, Moore, Weber, & Grant, 2009). This is because white matter injury is predominantly implicated in compromised processing speed (Anderson, 2002; McArthur, Brew, & Nath, 2005; Sarma et al., 2014). Research by Ackermann et al. (2016) found that despite early uptake of ART (4 months mean age), white matter changes were present in a sample of HIV-positive children (mean age 5) especially in the cortico-spinal tracts, but with less damage observed in the corpus callosum. In another study by Jankiewicz et al. (2017), the authors also found white matter changes in a sample of children (mean age 7) despite an early uptake of ART. The authors hypothesize that white matter injury occurs soon after infection. Even though the research focused on children, its findings are relevant to this study in that they illustrate the vulnerability of white matter to HIV infection. Ackermann et al. (2016) however assert that with continuous use of ART, HIV associated white matter injury can be contained.

In summary, the findings of the current study regarding the executive function domains - with the exception of processing speed (albeit only after the removal of outliers) - do not align with existing literature which evidences differences in scores of executive function tests between HIV-positive adolescents and controls (Laughton et al., 2013; Phillips et al., 2016). However, the present study findings are consistent with at least some other studies which have similarly found no differences in cognitive functioning between HIV-positive children and adolescents and matched controls (Blanchette, Smith, King, Fernandes-Penney, & Read, 2002; Dollfus et al., 2010). For example, a study of Ugandan children aged 6 to 12 years found no differences in cognitive performance of a sample of 28 prenatally-infected children, 42 children that were prenatally exposed but HIV-negative, and 37 HIV-negative controls. The three groups were matched for age and socioeconomic status. The study hypothesis was that the HIV-positive children would show more cognitive impairment relative to the other groups. However, their hypothesis was not confirmed in that study results revealed that the HIV-positive group performed within the expected age appropriate range of the cognitive tests used in that study (the study used the Kaufman Battery Assessment for Children – K-ABC). The authors explained that these findings were likely due to the HIV-positive children being asymptomatic due to a less aggressive disease progression. Although the aforementioned study is comparable to the present study in that it is also a SSA study, the participants' age range is dissimilar and also all participants in that study were ART naïve (not yet started on ART). Further, a Dutch study of 22 HIV- positive children and adolescents aged between 6 – 17 years revealed that they performed within national standards on psychomotor tests used in that study (Koekkoek et al., 2008). It was inferred in that study that the result may be a function of unsuitable measures of gross motor deficits.

Potential reasons for the non-significant between-group differences found in the current study are presented next. The first reason relates to reported restorative potential of ART on the CNS. A second consideration is with regards to social factors, which emerging literature reveals has profound negative implications on cognition that are separable from pathological mechanisms.

Explanations for non-significant between-group differences.

ART's protective properties on the CNS. The positive effects of ART on the CNS are widely reported in literature with most researchers attributing an unprecedented decline in the incidence of cognitive impairment and a marked decline in AIDS-related morbidity and mortality, to the introduction of ART (Brahmbhatt et al., 2014; Crowell et al., 2015; Heaton et al., 2011; Nachega et al., 2010; Spies et al., 2016; Willen et al., 2017; Williams et al., 2006). According to Llorente et al. (2014) ART not only protects the brain, but in some instances, may reverse HIV-related diseases in children. The benefits of ART are believed to stem fundamentally from ART's inherent predisposition to prevent viral replication, thus preserving the CNS from further HIV-associated impairment (Nichols et al., 2016). It is therefore plausible that the finding of non-significant between-group differences in the HIV-positive group and control group on neuropsychological test scores found in this study, reflect these mitigating effects of ART on the CNS. The result that 61% of the HIV-positive participants of this study had a low detectable viral load at the time of testing, is indicative of predominantly adherent patterns to ART in the HIV-positive group.

Notwithstanding the widely reported benefits of ART on cognition, it is also important to acknowledge an existing body of literature that counters this view and suggests that while taking up ART expands life expectancy, it does not always translate to positive effects on cognition (Heaton et al., 2011; Louthrenoo, Oberdorfer, & Sirisanthana, 2014; Spudich et al., 2019). For example, a study of Thai children established that ART uptake did not correspond to improvements in cognition even in children who had attained viral suppression (Puthanakit et al., 2010). Likewise, a local study by Hoare et al. (2016) of HIV-negative children and adolescents (*n* = 34) and HIV-positive children and adolescents (*n* = 86) aged 6 – 16 years found that despite being stably on ART, 45% of the HIV-positive children and adolescents had neurocognitive impairment and 18 adolescents in the HIV-positive group met the criteria for HIVE.

Notwithstanding inconsistent reports on the effectiveness of ART in reducing HIV-related morbidity and cognitive deficits, the bulk of the literature in this area, however, conveys convincing assertions in both international and local studies on the advantages of ART on the CNS. Still, emerging research is recognizing the role of environmental factors on cognition in the context of HIV and that these factors may confound an HIV presentation; one of these factors is social trauma.

Social trauma. Although there is a wide body of research on the impact of contextual factors on neurocognitive development, research focussing specifically on personal adverse experiences is gaining traction, particularly regarding the power of such experiences to undermine neurocognition and confound HIV-related neurocognitive effects. Specifically, there is increased acknowledgement in literature of the impact of childhood trauma on cognition and also how childhood trauma contributes to increased HIV risk behaviour and infection (Clark et al., 2012; Durevall & Lindskog, 2015; Fang, Chuang, & Lee, 2016; Senn, Carey, & Vanable, 2008).

An example of a study that highlights the detrimental impact of social trauma on the brain in the context of HIV and the resultant effects on neurocognition was conducted by Spies et al. (2016). The study was conducted in Cape Town, South Africa and included a sample of 124 HIV-positive women (age 18 - 65 years). Although conducted exclusively on older women the findings of the study are relevant to this study because the requirement of the study was that the reported trauma should have occurred before age 18 which incorporates the age range of this study's participants. Specifically, participants were screened for abuse and neglect. As part of the study design, the women were divided into 4 sub-groups: HIV-positive women that had experienced trauma early in life, HIV-positive women with no experienced trauma in their early life, HIV-negative women who had no early life trauma and, HIV-negative women who had experienced trauma early in their lives. The findings of the study revealed that the women who were dually affected by HIV and early life trauma had smaller brain volumes when compared to the other sub-groups. These abnormalities were especially pronounced on the corpus callosum, basal ganglia, limbic cortex (anterior cingulate cortex and amygdala) and hippocampi bilaterally. The brain alterations were conjectured to stem from the women's early life trauma and that they correlated with compromised cognitive performance particularly with regard to processing speed, working memory, abstraction and language ability. Essentially, relative to all of the study groups, the HIV-positive group with trauma performed the worst across the neurocognitive domains. Interestingly, the HIV-positive group with trauma performed comparatively to the HIV-negative group with trauma on attention, working memory and motor skills. Another notable finding of this study was that the HIV-positive group with no trauma performed similarly to the HIV-negative groups. In sum, it was only the addition of trauma that created a significant difference between the HIV-positive and HIV-negative groups on neurocognitive outcomes, with the HIV-positive groups with trauma performing the worst. These findings do perhaps question the role of trauma (or unaccounted for role in many cases) in studies that have reported significant differences in neurocognitive outcomes between HIV-positive and HIV-negative groups. Of course, social trauma was not assessed in the current study, so I cannot confidently comment on its effect relative to the current study results, but it does seem to be an emerging factor that should be considered in HIV research and may explain instances where non-significant between-group differences are found for HIV-positive and HIV-negative individuals.

Overall low executive function outcome scores for the two groups. As mentioned already, the executive function outcome scores of both the HIV-positive group and controls when compared to the normative scores of the tests used were low (by at least 2 SDs below the tests' means). These low scores suggest the presence of latent factors which influence cognition more generally, in the overall sample. Previous investigations into the impact of social factors on cognition reveal it to be not only profound but commonly negative (Boyede, Lesi, Ezeaka, & Umeh, 2013). Moreover, the negative effect of social factors on cognition has been found to present similarly, clinically, to fallout from pathological or neurological mechanisms (Fang et al., 2016, Natrass et al., 2012; Senn et al., 2008). Although social factors are wide-ranging (e.g., trauma, stigmatisation, food security, employment and education status) in this discussion I will focus on SES and quality of education.

Socioeconomic status (SES) and quality of education. SES is widely recognized in literature to impact negatively on cognitive development. So significant is the impact of SES on cognition that it often is demonstrable even in the absence of neurological impairment (Hackman, Gallop, Evans, & Farah, 2015; Jednoróg et al., 2012). Generally, a higher SES is associated with better cognitive functioning, while, low SES commonly represents poverty, limited education, malnutrition, poor medical access and poor mental stimulation, and is usually associated with poor cognitive functioning (Ferrett et al., 2014; Hackman et al., 2015; Hoare et al., 2016; Mosdell, Balchin, & Ameen, 2010). For instance, a study by Smith et al. (2013) in which they compared 3 groups of HIV-positive children and adolescents (7 -16 years) with a previous HIV disease, without a previous HIV disease, and prenatally-exposed but not infected, found that SES appeared to sub-serve differences in performance. In that study, whilst all 3 groups performed in the low average range cognitively, the children and adolescents who lived with their parents and were from families with higher income levels performed better on cognitive testing.

A related factor to SES is quality of education. Specifically, poor neuropsychological test outcomes have been shown to correlate with poor quality of education (Ferrett et al., 2014; Mosdell et al., 2010; Shuttleworth-Edwards et al., 2004; Shuttleworth-Edwards et al., 2013). Despite the collapse of the apartheid system of governance in South Africa, which apportioned resources according to race, disparities in resource allocation within the education sector have persisted well beyond the end of the apartheid regime (Ferrett et al., 2014; Mosdell et al., 2010). These disparities have repercussions on the quality of education offered in schools. Poor quality of education is typically associated with schools that are poorly resourced - in terms of both school supplies and personnel (e.g., lower qualified educators). Schools with high teacher/student ratios and those geographically located in areas where there are higher levels of crime tend to be associated with poor quality of education (Ferrett et al., 2014).

Consistent with this viewpoint, a study by Shuttleworth-Edwards et al. (2013) of South African learners from the Eastern Cape province (aged 12 – 13; $N = 69$) found that learners from advantaged schools outperformed learners from disadvantaged schools on cognitive testing by more than 10 scaled points. In that study, private and former Model C schools (which are predominantly English medium schools) were identified as advantaged schools and were associated with good quality of education. Disadvantaged schools which denoted poor quality of education were schools located in the townships; these schools were largely associated with under qualified teachers and a general lack of supplies and basic classroom resources such as school furniture. Using the WISC-IV, that study found that learners from advantaged schools fared superiorly to their peers from disadvantaged schools. For example, advantaged Black isiXhosa learners attained a mean FSIQ = 93.92 ($SD = 5.85$) compared to disadvantaged learners of the same race and age who attained a mean FSIQ = 77.08 ($SD = 13.79$). Given that the study had included neurological impairment as an exclusion criterion the study concluded that the key explanation for the vast discrepancy in performance were differences in quality of education. Consistent outcomes have been reported in previous studies of a similar nature (Shuttleworth-Jordan & Bode, 1995; Zindi, 2004).

Given that the participants in this study were predominantly from schools pegged at a low school quintile (i.e., school quintile 2), one may surmise that the participants came largely from poorly resourced schools which, as explained, are typically associated with poor quality of education. Given the reported relationship between neuropsychological test performance and poorer quality of education (Shuttleworth-Edwards et al., 2013), when considering the poor performance in the executive function tests of this study's participants, it is possible that the low executive function scores for both groups reflect the negative effects of these factors on neurocognitive development reported frequently in literature (Ferrett et al., 2014; Hackman et al., 2015; Hoare et al., 2016; Mosdell et al., 2010). It is therefore reasonable to contemplate that SES and poor quality of education may have had far more reaching implications for test performance on both groups and may have unduly hampered the performance of the participants. Related to SES, are methodological factors; research shows that using tests normed on Western populations in local contexts undermines their efficacy.

Methodological factors. In discussing the role of methodological factors in the attainment of low executive function scores for both groups, I will focus on the impact of non-local neuropsychological tests on performance.

One of the major critiques of the use of non-local neuropsychological tests in local settings is their apparent ineptitude in definitively discriminating performance from neurologically impaired and unimpaired individuals (Ferrett et al., 2014; Mosdell et al., 2010). Typically, when using these tests in local contexts, both impaired and unimpaired individuals can frequently be diagnosed as being impaired (Ferrett et al, 2014; Mosdell et al., 2010). The apparent failure of non-local neuropsychological tests to discriminate between neurologically and non-neurologically intact individuals, is because non-local neuropsychological tests are referenced on Western norms which differ markedly from those in developing countries (Ferrett et al., 2014). Norms are important because they are used as a reference against which an individual's performance is assessed and usually correspond to the contexts in which they are developed. The tests' norms used in this study are largely based on European and United States populations where the context is starkly different from South Africa in terms of SES, language and quality of education.

Furthermore, non-local neuropsychological tests appear to be more effective when administered on populations that have embraced a Western culture because Western acculturation parallels Western normative data (Ferrett et al, 2014; Manly, 2008; Mosdell et al., 2010). Secondly, a higher degree of Western acculturation is assumed to espouse better English language proficiency and quality of education both of which advantage one who is tested using non-local neuropsychological tests (Ferrett et al., 2014). Given that the participants in this study were not first language, English speakers and that they came from a predominantly non-western culture, it is possible that their attaining low executive function scores illustrates their limited western acculturation which may have unduly affected test performance resulting in lower scores than expected.

In sum, even though there was an isiXhosa translator present throughout testing, the influence of using tests that were designed and normed for western cultures on a predominantly non-western population may have impacted negatively on all of the current study participants' performance. It is possible that by using non-local tests the executive function scores of participants in this study may have been underestimated and therefore they may appear worse than they actually are (Shuttleworth-Jordan, 1996; Ferrett at al., 2014; Mosdell et al., 2010).

Aim 2: To Investigate Correlations Between Adherence and Executive Function

There is general consensus in literature that consistent adherence to ART is associated with improved cognitive outcomes. For example, a longitudinal study of HIV prenatally - infected children and adolescents by Crowell et al. (2015) found that ART uptake was positively correlated with improved neurocognitive outcomes. This finding was based on an analysis of two cohorts of the study – an earlier one that had poor access to ART (due to poor availability) and a second one which had a more consistent access to ART. A comparison of these cohorts revealed that children and adolescents who not only had earlier age uptake (age < 3) of ART, but also had regular access to ART, exhibited improved performance on cognitive testing for school-related tests than the cohort that had poor access to ART. The improvement in cognitive testing outcome was attributed to a more consistent access to ART.

Specific to the current study findings, the observed negative relationship between both cognitive flexibility and goal setting, and adherence, suggests that lower viral load (higher adherence) was associated with better cognitive flexibility and goal setting ability, albeit not significantly so. This finding, at least descriptively, is consistent with literature on HIV-related goal setting and cognitive flexibility difficulties and how poor adherence to ART may exacerbate impairment in these domains (Cattie et al., 2012; Laughton et al., 2013). The fact that the results in the current study were not significant could perhaps be explained by the lack of power, given the sample size. This outcome would be consistent with that reported by Nichols et al. (2012) of American adolescents aged 8-18 years ($N = 151$) who also found no correlation between cognitive functioning and adherence, but largely attributed this finding to their small sample size. Although that study is comparable to the present study regarding the age range, it however used pill count as a measurement of adherence.

In discordance with my hypothesis, the correlation between adherence and attentional control and information processing, although also not significant, was surprisingly positive, suggesting that a higher viral load (poor adherence) was associated with better attentional control and information processing. Given the pathophysiology of HIV, particularly its predilection for brain white matter and the fronto-striatal pathways, this finding is surprising (Abbott, Rönnbäck, & Hansson, 2006; Laughton et al., 2013; Smith & Wilkins, 2015; Thomas et al., 2016; Woods et al., 2009). This finding also stands in contrast with previous literature which determined that poor adherence is negatively associated with attentional control and the speed at which information is processed (Fellows et al., 2014; Wood, Shah, Steenhoff, & Rutstein, 2009).

It is unclear why the correlations between adherence and the executive function composites were not significant and why the correlations between attentional control and processing speed and adherence were positive, particularly since it is widely theorized in literature that higher adherence to ART is associated with improved neurocognition (see Hudelson & Cluver, 2015; Nachega et al., 2014; Peltzer & Pengpid, 2013). It may well be that these unexpected findings are a result of the study being underpowered, as previously alluded to.

A second plausible explanation worth considering for these unexpected findings may relate to statistical analyses limitations pertaining to the adherence (viral load) data. To explain, the adherence data (viral load) for participants used in this study is archival or retrospective data that was collected from patient medical files at Hannan Crusaid clinic. This is because procedurally the Hannan Crusaid clinic in partnership with the Desmond Tutu HIV Foundation does not regularly measure viral load, rather, viral load is typically measured when participants start to exhibit symptoms of opportunistic infections (Dr. M. Atujuna, personal communication, October 2018). Therefore, it is likely that the varied time points in viral load measurement and the collection of participant neuropsychological data may have introduced vast variance in the data thus introducing the risk of violating the normal distribution principle (Fields, 2009). Although the adherence data was statistically transformed by introducing a log function to reduce possible impact of variance, potential effects of variance in the analysis cannot be completely discounted.

A third probable explanation for the study findings relates to cerebral spinal fluid (CSF) escape. CSF escape is defined as detected CSF viral load when the plasma viral load reflects an undetectable level by the same laboratory assay used in measuring the plasma viral load (Collier et al., 2018). Essentially, this suggests that an undetectable plasma HIV reading may at times mask a detectable CSF HIV load which implies that virologically suppressed individuals may have detectable CSF viral loads (Collier et al., 2018; Letendre, 2011). The mechanism for CSF escape is unclear, however there is postulation that it may have to do with the difficulty of some ARVs to effectively cross the BBB (Letendre, 2011; Spudich et al., 2019). As previously mentioned, the BBB forms a protective barrier around the brain that obstructs the passage of toxic substances into the brain parenchyma (Collier et al., 2018; Smith & Wilkins, 2015). Unfortunately, in carrying out this function, the BBB may block the passage of some types of ARVs (Letendre, 2011; Spudich et al., 2019). When the BBB blocks the passage of some types of ARVs, it can effectively lead to the creation of a protected environment or reservoir for HIV in the brain, in which the virus continues to replicate without ARV drug mitigation (Letendre, 2011).

Finally, given that the current study utilized plasma viral load readings to evaluate adherence it is reasonable to speculate that these do not sufficiently account for CSF viral load levels, which may well be discordant to the plasma readings. Importantly, this reasoning may partially explain the contradiction reflected in the adherence data and executive function composite correlation coefficients derived in the current study.

Limitations and Recommendations

Despite taking care to ensure that this study was methodically and conceptually sound, this study is not without limitations. The results should thus be considered with these in mind.

Firstly, the small sample size calls for a cautious interpretation of the results. A post hoc analysis revealed that given the sample size with two groups ($N = 44$), using an alpha level of .05 and a medium effect size of Cohen's $d = 0.50$, a statistical power of 0.49 was generated. This means the study is underpowered and therefore future studies should consider increasing the sample size. The study sample size was impacted by unforeseen delays in the finalisation of amendments to the ethical protocol of the larger HlangananiPlus HCT project, which necessitated a delay in the commencement of the larger project. Given that this study drew its HIV-positive participants from the larger project, the delays encountered in the larger project had repercussions on the timeline of the present study especially regarding its commencement. The requirement was that all testing of participants of the current study had to be completed before the start of the HlanagananiPlus HCT project to prevent participant fatigue and to ensure availability of participants for the activities and tasks of the larger project. I managed to test 22 HIV-positive participants prior the commencement of the larger study.

A second limitation to the study is that my analyses of executive function did not include measures of all the sub-components of the four domains outlined in P. Anderson's (2002) executive function framework on which my analyses is based (e.g., feedback utilisation, self-regulation, efficiency and initiative). Including measures for all the sub-components may have produced a more comprehensive analysis.

A third limitation to the study is that it did not sufficiently assess social factors, specifically personal trauma and a broader description of participants' SES. Social factors, as discussed, are known to have profound impact on neurocognition to the extent that they can mimic neurological fallout even in the absence of pathology (Hackman et al., 2015). Although school quintile is an informative index to gauge SES level, it is limited in effectively assessing SES in the sense that it does not comprehensively represent the different elements of SES such as family income, family asset base and level of education of parents (Falagas, Zarkadoulia, Pliatsika, & Panos, 2008; Peltzer & Pengpid, 2013). Therefore, future studies should seek to acquire a comprehensive social profile of participants. In the current study, as mentioned, a demographic and asset index questionnaire was distributed for caregivers to complete but due to poor completion and return rates the information could not be utilised in this study.

Fourthly, the study did not undertake a comprehensive behavioural assessment of the sample in the study which would have provided more insight into the executive presentation of the adolescents. This is in the sense that there are behavioural components to executive function that cannot be exclusively nor accurately demonstrated by pencil and paper cognitive tests (Reisner et al., 2009). Additionally, developmentally, adolescents appear disproportionately more inclined to behavioural risk taking and engaging in activities considered HIV risk behaviours which has implications for executive function and adherence (Romer et al., 2017). Although the Behavioural Rating Inventory of Executive Function (BRIEF) and Child Behaviour Checklist and Youth Self Report were distributed as part of the current study, which are instruments aimed at collecting data on the behavioural components of executive functions, in the end this data was not used due to poor completion and return rates. Accordingly, future studies ought to include comprehensive evaluations of the behavioural profiles of adolescents from their standpoint as well as reports from caregivers for a balanced perspective to gain a more holistic picture of adolescent's cognitive presentation especially in their daily living. Poor return rates of this form of data is well documented in the literature (e.g., Land & Ross, 2014).

A fifth limitation of the current study is the use of self-reports and not a biomarker for establishing an HIV diagnosis for the HIV-negative controls. Although using self-reports to establish HIV status is prone to inaccuracies, this method is still widely used in research (e.g., Kufa et al., 2018; Rohr et al., 2017; Vannable et al., 2009).

Conclusion

The impact of HIV on cognition is profound, especially on a developing adolescent brain. Even though cognitive outcomes associated with HIV are wide-ranging, executive dysfunction is particularly rife among HIV-positive adolescents. Although the introduction of ART is reported to mitigate the effects of HIV on cognition, including executive dysfunction, significant differences in executive functioning between HIV-positive and HIV-negative adolescents are still widely reported in literature with HIV-positive adolescents performing more poorly than HIV-negative peers. The difference in performance is invariably attributed to HIV-related insult to the brain. However, emerging research suggests that these effects of HIV on cognition are confounded by social factors, that research does not often take into account, and which may explain outcomes where no significant differences are found between HIV-positive and HIV-negative participants. Understanding the role of these factors, alongside the potential mitigating effects of ARVs in explaining HIV outcomes, is important. Given the important role of ARVs in managing the effects of HIV, investigating factors that support or may undermine those effects are important. Although the findings in the current study did not conclusively provide evidence for the role of executive functions in adherence, further studies with larger samples should confirm such outcomes.

The current study adds to a growing body of knowledge on the impact of HIV on adolescent executive functioning. Considering that there is a paucity of research that focusses specifically on this group, and an even greater dearth of literature on executive function outcomes specifically on this high-risk population in terms of contracting HIV, the current study is timely. This is in the sense that a few studies have specifically investigated executive functions in a controlled trial of this nature; therefore, the findings of the present study are especially important as they add to emerging research of this nature.

References

Abbott, N. J., Rönnbäck, L., & Hansson, E. (2006). Astrocyte-endothelial interactions at the blood-brain barrier. *Nature Reviews Neuroscience*. https://doi.org/10.1038/nrn1824

Ackermann, C., Andronikou, S., Saleh, M. G., Laughton, B., Alhamud, A. A., Van Der Kouwe, A., … Meintjes, E. M. (2016). Early antiretroviral therapy in HIV-infected children is associated with diffuse white matter structural abnormality and corpus callosum sparing. *American Journal of Neuroradiology*, *37*(12), 2363–2369. https://doi.org/10.3174/ajnr.A4921

Anderson, P. (2002). Assessment and development of executive function (EF) during childhood. *Child Neuropsychology*. https://doi.org/10.1076/chin.8.2.71.8724

Anderson, V. A., Anderson, P., Northam, E., Jacobs, R., & Catroppa, C. (2001). Development of executive functions through late childhood and adolescence in an Australian sample. *Developmental Neuropsychology*. https://doi.org/10.1207/S15326942DN2001_5

Antinori, A., Heaton, R. K., & Marder, K. (2007). *Updated research nosology for HIV-associated neurocognitive disorders*.

Baufeldt, A. (2009). The effects of education on phonemic verbal fluency performance: An original empirical study and meta-analysis (Honours book). Retrieved from http://www.psychology.uct.ac.za/sites/default/files/image_tool/images/117/Angela.Baufeldt.pdf

Blanchette, N., Smith, M. Lou, King, S., Fernandes-Penney, A., & Read, S. (2002). Cognitive development in school-age children with vertically transmitted HIV infection. *Developmental Neuropsychology*. https://doi.org/10.1207/S15326942DN2103_1

Boivin, M. J., Barlow-Mosha, L., Chernoff, M. C., Laughton, B., Zimmer, B., Joyce, C., … Palumbo, P. E. (2018). Neuropsychological performance in African children with HIV enrolled in a multisite antiretroviral clinical trial. *AIDS*, *32*(2), 189–204. https://doi.org/10.1097/QAD.0000000000001683

Boyede, G. O., Lesi, F. E. A., Ezeaka, V. C., & Umeh, C. S. (2013). Impact of sociodemographic factors on cognitive function in school-aged HIV-infected Nigerian children. *HIV/AIDS - Research and Palliative Care*. https://doi.org/10.2147/HIV.S43260

Brahmbhatt, H., Boivin, M., Ssempijja, V., Kigozi, G., Kagaayi, J., Serwadda, D., & Gray, R. H. (2014). Neurodevelopmental benefits of antiretroviral therapy in ugandan children aged 0-6 years with HIV. *Journal of Acquired Immune Deficiency Syndromes*, *67*(3), 316–322. https://doi.org/10.1097/QAI.0000000000000295

Brydges, C. R., Reid, C. L., Fox, A. M., & Anderson, M. (2012). A unitary executive function predicts intelligence in children. *Intelligence*, *40*(5), 458–469. https://doi.org/10.1016/j.intell.2012.05.006

Cattie, J. E., Doyle, K., Weber, E., Grant, I., & Woods, S. P. (2012). Planning deficits in HIV-associated neurocognitive disorders: Component processes, cognitive correlates, and implications for everyday functioning. *Journal of Clinical and Experimental Neuropsychology*, *34*(9), 906–918. https://doi.org/10.1080/13803395.2012.692772

Chesney, M. A. (2000). Factors Affecting Adherence to Antiretroviral Therapy. *Clinical Infectious Diseases*. https://doi.org/10.1086/313849

Chiriboga, C. A., Fleishman, S., Champion, S., Gaye-Robinson, L., & Abrams, E. J. (2005). Incidence and prevalence of HIV encephalopathy in children with HIV infection receiving highly active anti-retroviral therapy (HAART). *Journal of Pediatrics*. https://doi.org/10.1016/j.jpeds.2004.10.021

Clark, U., Cohen, R., Sweet, L., Gongvatana, A., Devlin, K., Hana, G., . . . Tashima, K. (2012). Effects of HIV and Early Life Stress on Amygdala Morphometry and Neurocognitive Function. *Journal of the International Neuropsychological Society*, *18*(4), 657-668. doi:10.1017/S1355617712000434

Cohen, M. (1997). Children's memory scale (CMS). *San Antonio: The Psychological Corporation.*

Cohen, S., Caan, M. W. A., Mutsaerts, H. J., Scherpbier, H. J., Kuijpers, T. W., Reiss, P., … Pajkrt, D. (2016). Cerebral injury in perinatally HIV-infected children compared to matched healthy controls. *Neurology*, *86*(1), 19–27. https://doi.org/10.1212/WNL.0000000000002209

Cohen, S., Ter Stege, J. A., Geurtsen, G. J., Scherpbier, H. J., Kuijpers, T. W., Reiss, P., … Pajkrt, D. (2015). Poorer cognitive performance in perinatally HIV-infected children versus healthy socioeconomically matched controls. *Clinical Infectious Diseases*, *60*(7), 1111–1119. https://doi.org/10.1093/cid/ciu1144

Collier, D. A., Haddow, L., Brijkumar, J., Moosa, M. Y. S., Benjamin, L., & Gupta, R. K. (2018). HIV cerebrospinal fluid escape and neurocognitive pathology in the era of combined antiretroviral therapy: What lies beneath the tip of the Iceberg in Sub-Saharan Africa? *Brain Sciences*, Vol. 8. https://doi.org/10.3390/brainsci8100190

Cross, H. M., Combrinck, M. I., & Joska, J. A. (2013). HIV-associated neurocognitive disorders: Antiretroviral regimen, central nervous system penetration effectiveness, and cognitive outcomes. *South African Medical Journal*. https://doi.org/10.7196/SAMJ.6677

Crowell, C. S., Huo, Y., Tassiopoulos, K., Malee, K. M., Yogev, R., Hazra, R., … Muller, W. J. (2015). Early viral suppression improves neurocognitive outcomes in HIV-infected children. *AIDS*, *29*(3), 295–304. https://doi.org/10.1097/QAD.0000000000000528

Delis, D. C., Kaplan, E., & Kramer, J. H. (2001). Delis-Kaplan executive function scale. . *San Antonio, TX: The Psychological Corporation.* https://doi.org/10.3109/02770903.2012.715704

Department of Basic Education. (2018). School Masterlist Data. Retrieved from https://www.education.gov.za/EMIS/EMISDownloads/tabid/466/Default.aspx

Desmond Tutu HIV Research Foundation. (2017). Retaining HIV-positive youth in care: A model for transitioning adolescents receiving ART from pediatric to adult care. (Unpublished project protocol). Cape Town, South Africa.

Diamond, A. (2013). Executive Functions. *Annual Review of Psychology*. https://doi.org/10.1146/annurev-psych-113011-143750

Dollfus, C., Le Chenadec, J., Faye, A., Blanche, S., Briand, N., Rouzioux, C., & Warszawski, J. (2010). Long-Term Outcomes in Adolescents Perinatally Infected with HIV-1 and Followed Up since Birth in the French Perinatal Cohort (EPF/ANRS CO10). *Clinical Infectious Diseases*, *51*(2), 214–224. https://doi.org/10.1086/653674

Donald, K. A., Walker, K. G., Kilborn, T., Carrara, H., Langerak, N. G., Eley, B., & Wilmshurst, J. M. (2015). HIV Encephalopathy: Pediatric case series description and insights from the clinic coalface. *AIDS Research and Therapy*. https://doi.org/10.1186/s12981-014-0042-7

Dumontheil, I. (2015). Desarrollo del cerebro social durante la adolescencia. *Psicologia Educativa*, *21*(2), 117–124. https://doi.org/10.1016/j.pse.2015.08.001

Durevall, D., & Lindskog, A. (2015). Intimate Partner Violence and HIV Infection in sub-Saharan Africa. *World Development*, *72*, 27–42. https://doi.org/10.1016/j.worlddev.2015.02.012

Esbjörnsson, J., Månsson, F., Kvist, A., da Silva, Z. J., Andersson, S., Fenyö, E. M., … Wilhelmson, S. (2019). Long-term follow-up of HIV-2-related AIDS and mortality in Guinea-Bissau: a prospective open cohort study. *The Lancet HIV*, *6*(1), e25–e31. https://doi.org/10.1016/S2352-3018(18)30254-6

Falagas, M. E., Zarkadoulia, E. A., Pliatsika, P. A., & Panos, G. (2008). Socioeconomic status (SES) as a determinant of adherence to treatment in HIV infected patients: A systematic review of the literature. *Retrovirology*. https://doi.org/10.1186/1742-4690-5-13

Fang, L., Chuang, D. M., & Lee, Y. (2016). Adverse childhood experiences, gender, and HIV risk behaviors: Results from a population-based sample. *Preventive Medicine Reports*, *4*, 113–120. https://doi.org/10.1016/j.pmedr.2016.05.019

Fellows, R. P., Byrd, D. A., & Morgello, S. (2014). Effects of information processing speed on learning, memory, and executive functioning in people living with HIV/AIDS. *Journal of Clinical and Experimental Neuropsychology*. https://doi.org/10.1080/13803395.2014.943696

Ferrett, H. L., Carey, P. D., Thomas, K. G. F., Tapert, S. F., & Fein, G. (2010). Neuropsychological performance of South African treatment-naïve adolescents with alcohol dependence. *Drug and Alcohol Dependence*. https://doi.org/10.1016/j.drugalcdep.2010.01.019

Ferrett, H. L. (2011). The Adaptation and Norming of Selected Psychometric Tests for 12- to 15-year-old Urbanized Western Cape Adolescents (Doctoral book). Retrieved from

https://pdfs.semanticscholar.org/95b1/cb95c2e6368e9d7c391ddce7764feb703566.pdf

Ferrett, H. L., Thomas, K. G. F., Tapert, S. F., Carey, P. D., Conradie, S., Cuzen, N. L., … Fein, G. (2014). The cross-cultural utility of foreign- and locally-derived normative data for three WHO-endorsed neuropsychological tests for South African adolescents. *Metabolic Brain Disease*, *29*(2), 395–408. https://doi.org/10.1007/s11011-014-9495-6

Field, A. (2009). Exploring assumptions. In *Discovering Statistics Using SPSS*. https://doi.org/10.1111/insr.12011_21

Fraser, S. (2013). Memory functioning in HIV positive adolescents receiving anti-retroviral treatment (Doctoral book). Retrieved from wiredspace.wits.ac.za

Fujiwara, E., Tomlinson, S. E., Purdon, S. E., Gill, M. J., & Power, C. (2015). Decision making under explicit risk is impaired in individuals with human immunodeficiency virus (HIV). *Journal of Clinical and Experimental Neuropsychology*, *37*(7), 733–750. https://doi.org/10.1080/13803395.2015.1057481

Giacomet, V., Albano, F., Starace, F., De Franciscis, A., Giaquinto, C., Castelli Gattinara, G., … Guarino, A. (2003). Adherence to antiretroviral therapy and its determinants in children with human immunodeficiency virus infection: A multicentre, national study. *Acta Paediatrica, International Journal of Paediatrics*. https://doi.org/10.1080/08035250310006737

Global AIDS Monitoring. (2018). Indicators for monitoring the 2016 United Nations Political Declaration on Ending AIDS. Retrieved from https://www.unaids.org/sites/default/files/media_asset/2017-Global-AIDS-Monitoring_en.pdf

Hackman, D. A., Gallop, R., Evans, G. W., & Farah, M. J. (2015). Socioeconomic status and executive function: Developmental trajectories and mediation. *Developmental Science*. https://doi.org/10.1111/desc.12246

Hammond, C. K., Eley, B., & Wilmshurst, J. M. (2019). Neuropsychiatric and Neurocognitive Manifestations in HIV-infected Children Treated with Efavirenz in South Africa–A Retrospective Case Series. *Frontiers in Neurology, 10,* 742.

Heaton, R. K., Franklin, D. R., Deutsch, R., Letendre, S., Ellis, R. J., Casaletto, K., … Grant, I. (2015). Neurocognitive change in the era of HIV combination antiretroviral therapy: The longitudinal CHARTER study. *Clinical Infectious Diseases*, *60*(3), 473–480. https://doi.org/10.1093/cid/ciu862

Heaton, R. K., Franklin, D. R., Ellis, R. J., McCutchan, J. A., Letendre, S. L., LeBlanc, S., … Grant, I. (2011). HIV-associated neurocognitive disorders before and during the era of combination antiretroviral therapy: Differences in rates, nature, and predictors. *Journal of NeuroVirology*, *17*(1), 3–16. https://doi.org/10.1007/s13365-010-0006-1

Hermetet-Lindsay, K. D., Correia, K. F., Williams, P. L., Smith, R., Malee, K. M., Mellins, C. A., & Rutstein, R. M. (2017). Contributions of Disease Severity, Psychosocial Factors, and Cognition to Behavioral Functioning in US Youth Perinatally Exposed to HIV. *AIDS and Behavior*, *21*(9), 2703–2715. https://doi.org/10.1007/s10461-016-1508-5

Hinkin, C. H., Hardy, D. J., Mason, K. I., Castellon, S. A., Durvasula, R. S., Lam, M. N., & Stefaniak, M. (2004). Medication adherence in HIV-infected adults: effect of patient age, cognitive status, and substance abuse. AIDS (London, England), 18 Suppl 1(Suppl 1), S19–S25. doi:10.1097/00002030-200418001-00004

Hoare, J., Phillips, N., Joska, J. A., Paul, R., Donald, K. A., Stein, D. J., & Thomas, K. G. F. (2016). Applying the HIV-associated neurocognitive disorder diagnostic criteria to HIV-infected youth. *Neurology*, *87*(1), 86–93. https://doi.org/10.1212/WNL.0000000000002669

Hudelson, C., & Cluver, L. (2015). Factors associated with adherence to antiretroviral therapy among adolescents living with HIV/AIDS in low- and middle-income countries: A systematic review. *AIDS Care - Psychological and Socio-Medical Aspects of AIDS/HIV*, *27*(7), 805–816. https://doi.org/10.1080/09540121.2015.1011073

Inzaule, S. C., Hamers, R. L., Kityo, C., Rinke De Wit, T. F., & Roura, M. (2016). Long-term antiretroviral treatment adherence in HIV-infected adolescents and adults in Uganda: A qualitative study. *PLoS ONE*. https://doi.org/10.1371/journal.pone.0167492

Jacobs, G. B., Loxton, A. G., Laten, A., Robson, B., Janse Van Rensburg, E., & Engelbrecht, S. (2009). Emergence and diversity of different HIV-1 subtypes in South Africa, 2000-2001. *Journal of Medical Virology*. https://doi.org/10.1002/jmv.21609

Jankiewicz, M., Holmes, M. J., Taylor, P. A., Cotton, M. F., Laughton, B., van der Kouwe, A. J. W., & Meintjes, E. M. (2017). White matter abnormalities in children with HIV infection and exposure. *Frontiers in Neuroanatomy*, *11*. https://doi.org/10.3389/fnana.2017.00088

Jednoróg, K., Altarelli, I., Monzalvo, K., Fluss, J., Dubois, J., Billard, C., … Ramus, F. (2012). The influence of socioeconomic status on children's brain structure. *PLoS ONE*. https://doi.org/10.1371/journal.pone.0042486

Joska, J. A., Westgarth-Taylor, J., Myer, L., Hoare, J., Thomas, K. G. F., Combrinck, M., … Flisher, A. J. (2011). Characterization of HIV-Associated Neurocognitive Disorders among individuals starting antiretroviral therapy in South Africa. *AIDS and Behavior*, *15*(6), 1197–1203. https://doi.org/10.1007/s10461-010-9744-6

Kim, S. H., Gerver, S. M., Fidler, S., & Ward, H. (2014). Adherence to antiretroviral therapy in adolescents living with HIV: Systematic review and meta-analysis. *Aids*, *28*(13), 1945–1956. https://doi.org/10.1097/QAD.0000000000000316

Koekkoek, S., de Sonneville, L. M. J., Wolfs, T. F. W., Licht, R., & Geelen, S. P. M. (2008). Neurocognitive function profile in HIV-infected school-age children. *European Journal of Paediatric Neurology*, *12*(4), 290–297. https://doi.org/10.1016/j.ejpn.2007.09.002

Korkman, M., Kirk, U., & Kemp, S. (2007). Design and Purpose of the NEPSY-II. *The NEPSY.*

Kufa, T., Maseko, V. D., Nhlapo, D., Radebe, F., Puren, A., & Kularatne, R. S. (2018). Knowledge of HIV status and antiretroviral therapy use among sexually transmitted infections service attendees and the case for improving the integration of services in South Africa A cross sectional study. *Medicine (United States)*, *97*(39), 1–8. https://doi.org/10.1097/MD.0000000000012575

Kwak, S. K., & Kim, J. H. (2017). Statistical data preparation: management of missing values and outliers. Korean journal of anesthesiology, 70(4), 407. doi: 10.4097/kjae.2017.70.4.407

Land, L., Ross, J. D. (2014). Barriers to questionnaire completion: understanding the AIDS/HIV patient's perspective. *Nurse Res,21*(3), 20–3, DOI: 10.7748/nr2014.01.21.3.20.e1227

Laughton, B., Cornell, M., Boivin, M., & Van Rie, A. (2013). Neurodevelopment in perinatally HIV-infected children: a concern for adolescence. *Journal of the International AIDS Society*, *16*(1), 18603. https://doi.org/10.7448/IAS.16.1.18603

Laurikkala, J., Juhola, M., Kentala, E., Lavrac, N., Miksch, S., & Kavsek, B. (2000, August). Informal identification of outliers in medical data. In Fifth international workshop on intelligent data analysis in medicine and pharmacology, l, 20-24.

Letendre, S. (2011). Central nervous system complications in HIV disease: HIV-associated neurocognitive disorder. *Topics in Antiviral Medicine*, *19*(4), 137–142.

Lewis-de los Angeles, C. P., Williams, P. L., Huo, Y., Wang, S. D., Uban, K. A., Herting, M. M., … Wang, L. (2017). Lower total and regional grey matter brain volumes in youth with perinatally-acquired HIV infection: Associations with HIV disease severity, substance use, and cognition. *Brain, Behavior, and Immunity*, *62*, 100–109. https://doi.org/10.1016/j.bbi.2017.01.004

Llorente, A. M., Brouwers, P., Leighty, R., Malee, K., Smith, R., Harris, L., … Chase, C. (2014). An Analysis of Select Emerging Executive Skills in Perinatally HIV-1-Infected Children. *Applied Neuropsychology: Child*, *3*(1), 10–25. https://doi.org/10.1080/21622965.2012.686853

Llorente, A. M., Voigt, R. G., Williams, J., Frailey, J. K., Satz, P., & D'Elia, L. F. (2009). Children's color trails test 1 2: Test-retest reliability and factorial validity. *Clinical Neuropsychologist*. https://doi.org/10.1080/13854040802427795

Louthrenoo, O., Oberdorfer, P., & Sirisanthana, V. (2014). Psychosocial functioning in adolescents with perinatal HIV infection receiving highly active antiretroviral therapy. *Journal of the International Association of Providers of AIDS Care*, *13*(2), 178–183. https://doi.org/10.1177/2325957413488171

Malee, K., Williams, P. L., Montepiedra, G., Nichols, S., Sirois, P. A., Storm, D., … Team, P. (2009). *The Role of Cognitive Functioning in Medication Adherence of Children and Adolescents with HIV Infection*. *34*(2), 164–175.

Manly, J. J. (2008). Critical issues in cultural neuropsychology: Profit from diversity. *Neuropsychology Review*, *18*(3 SPEC. ISS.), 179–183. https://doi.org/10.1007/s11065-008-9068-8

Margot, N., Koontz, D., McCallister, S., Mellors, J. W., & Callebaut, C. (2018). Measurement of plasma HIV-1 RNA below the limit of quantification (<20 copies/mL) of commercial assays with the integrase HIV RNA single-copy assay. *Journal of Clinical Virology*, *108*(March), 50–52. https://doi.org/10.1016/j.jcv.2018.09.003

Mattson, S. N., Crocker, N., & Nguyen, T. T. (2011). Fetal alcohol spectrum disorders: Neuropsychological and behavioral features. *Neuropsychology Review*. https://doi.org/10.1007/s11065-011-9167-9

McArthur, J. C., Brew, B. J., & Nath, A. (2005). Neurological complications of HIV infection. *Lancet Neurology*. https://doi.org/10.1016/S1474-4422(05)70165-4

Medina, K. L., Hanson, K. L., Schweinsburg, A. D., Cohen-Zion, M., Nagel, B. J., & Tapert, S. F. (2007). Neuropsychological functioning in adolescent marijuana users: subtle deficits detectable after a month of abstinence. Journal of the International Neuropsychological Society: JINS, 13(5), 807–820. doi:10.1017/S1355617707071032

Mitchell, C. D. (2006). HIV-1 Encephalopathyamong Perinatally Infected Children: Neuropathogenisis and Response to HighlyActive Antiretroviral Therapy. *Mental Retardation and Developmnetal Disabilities Research Review, 12*(3), 216-222.

Mosdell, J., Balchin, R., & Ameen, O. (2010a). Adaptation of aphasia tests for neurocognitive screening in South Africa. *South African Journal of Psychology*, *40*(3), 250–261. https://doi.org/10.1177/008124631004000304

Mosdell, J., Balchin, R., & Ameen, O. (2010b). Adaptation of aphasia tests for neurocognitive screening in South Africa. *South African Journal of Psychology*, *40*(3), 250–261.

Nachega, J. B., Stein, D. M., Lehman, D. A., Hlatshwayo, D., Mothopeng, R., Chaisson, R. E., & Karstaedt, A. S. (2004). Adherence to antiretroviral therapy in HIV-infected adults in Soweto, South Africa. *AIDS Research and Human Retroviruses*. https://doi.org/10.1089/aid.2004.20.1053

Nachega, Jean B., Mills, E. J., & Schechter, M. (2010). Antiretroviral therapy adherence and retention in care in middle-income and low-income countries: Current status of knowledge and research priorities. *Current Opinion in HIV and AIDS*. https://doi.org/10.1097/COH.0b013e328333ad61

Nachega, Jean B., Uthman, O. A., Del Rio, C., Mugavero, M. J., Rees, H., & Mills, E. J. (2014). Addressing the achilles' heel in the HIV care continuum for the success of a test-and-treat strategy to achieve an AIDS-free generation. *Clinical Infectious Diseases*. https://doi.org/10.1093/cid/ciu299

Nagarajan, R., Sarma, M. K., Thomas, M. A., Chang, L., Natha, U., Wright, M., … Keller, M. A. (2012). Neuropsychological function and cerebral metabolites in HIV-infected youth. *Journal of Neuroimmune Pharmacology*. https://doi.org/10.1007/s11481-012-9407-7

Nichols, S. L., Brummel, S. S., Smith, R. A., Garvie, P. A., Hunter, S. J., Malee, K. M., … Willen, E. (2015). Executive Functioning in Children and Adolescents With Perinatal HIV Infection. *Pediatric Infectious Disease Journal*, *34*(9), 969–975. https://doi.org/10.1097/INF.0000000000000809

Nichols, S. L., Chernoff, M. C., Malee, K. M., Sirois, P. A., Woods, S. P., Williams, P. L., … Kammerer, B. (2016). Executive functioning in children and adolescents with perinatal HIV infection and perinatal HIV exposure. *Journal of the Pediatric Infectious Diseases Society*, *5*, S15–S23. https://doi.org/10.1093/jpids/piw049

Nichols, S. L., Montepiedra, G., Farley, J. J., Sirois, P. A., Malee, K., Kammerer, B., … Naar-King, S. (2012). Cognitive, academic, and behavioral correlates of medication adherence in children and adolescents with perinatally acquired HIV infection. *Journal of Developmental and Behavioral Pediatrics*, *33*(4), 298–308. https://doi.org/10.1097/DBP.0b013e31824bef47

Noble, K. G., Houston, S. M., Brito, N. H., Bartsch, H., Kan, E., Kuperman, J. M., … Sowell, E. R. (2015). Family income, parental education and brain structure in children and adolescents. *Nature Neuroscience*, *18*(5), 773–778. https://doi.org/10.1038/nn.3983

Nyamweya, S., Hegedus, A., Jaye, A., Rowland-Jones, S., Flanagan, K. L., & Macallan, D. C. (2013). Comparing HIV-1 and HIV-2 infection: Lessons for viral immunopathogenesis. *Reviews in Medical Virology*, Vol. 23, pp. 221–240. https://doi.org/10.1002/rmv.1739

Onyebujoh, P. C., Ribeiro, I., & Whalen, C. C. (2007). Treatment Options for HIV-Associated Tuberculosis. *The Journal of Infectious Diseases*, *196*(s1), S35–S45. https://doi.org/10.1086/518657

Peltzer, K., & Pengpid, S. (2013). Socioeconomic factors in adherence to HIV therapy in low- and middle-income countries. *Journal of Health, Population and Nutrition*. https://doi.org/10.3329/jhpn.v31i2.16379

Phillips, N., Amos, T., Kuo, C., Hoare, J., Ipser, J., F Thomas, K. G., & Stein, D. J. (2016). HIV-Associated Cognitive Impairment in Perinatally Infected Children: A Meta-analysis. In *Review Article PediatricS* (Vol. 138).

Phillips, N. J., Hoare, J., Stein, D. J., Myer, L., Zar, H. J., & Thomas, K. G. F. (2018). HIV-associated cognitive disorders in perinatally infected children and adolescents: a novel composite cognitive domains score. *AIDS Care - Psychological and Socio-Medical Aspects of AIDS/HIV*, *30*, 8–16. https://doi.org/10.1080/09540121.2018.1466982

Puthanakit, T., Aurpibul, L., Louthrenoo, O., Tapanya, P., Nadsasarn, R., Insee-Ard, S., &

Sirisanthana, V. (2010). Poor cognitive functioning of school-aged children in thailand with perinatally acquired HIV infection taking antiretroviral therapy. *AIDS Patient Care and STDs*, *24*(3), 141–146. https://doi.org/10.1089/apc.2009.0314

Reisner, S. L., Mimiaga, M. J., Skeer, M., Perkovich, B., Johnson, C. V., & Safren, S. A. (2009). A review of HIV antiretroviral adherence and intervention studies among HIV-infected youth. *Topics in HIV Medicine : A Publication of the International AIDS Society, USA*.

Rice, J., Correia, A. F., & Schutte, E. (2014). Attention and concentration functions in HIV-positive adolescents who are on anti-retroviral treatment. *South African Journal of Psychology*. https://doi.org/10.1177/0081246314540141

Rohr, J. K., Xavier Gómez-Olivé, F., Rosenberg, M., Manne-Goehler, J., Geldsetzer, P., Wagner, R. G., … Bärnighausen, T. (2017). Performance of self-reported HIV status in determining true HIV status among older adults in rural South Africa: A validation study: A. *Journal of the International AIDS Society*, *20*(1), 11–13. https://doi.org/10.7448/IAS.20.1.21691

Romer, D., Reyna, V. F., & Satterthwaite, T. D. (2017). Beyond stereotypes of adolescent risk taking: Placing the adolescent brain in developmental context. *Developmental Cognitive Neuroscience*, *27*(July), 19–34. https://doi.org/10.1016/j.dcn.2017.07.007

Ruel, T. D., Boivin, M. J., Boal, H. E., Bangirana, P., Charlebois, E., Havlir, D. V., … Wong, J. K. (2012). Neurocognitive and motor deficits in HIV-infected ugandan children with high CD4 cell counts. *Clinical Infectious Diseases*, *54*(7), 1001–1009. https://doi.org/10.1093/cid/cir1037

Saberi, P., Mayer, K., Vittinghoff, E., & Naar-King, S. (2014). Correlation Between Use of Antiretroviral Adherence Devices by HIV-Infected Youth and Plasma HIV RNA and Self-Reported Adherence. *AIDS and Behavior*, *19*(1), 93–103. https://doi.org/10.1007/s10461-014-0806-z

Santos, A. F., & Soares, M. A. (2010). HIV genetic diversity and drug resistance. *Viruses*, *2*(2), 503–531. https://doi.org/10.3390/v2020503

Sarma, M. K., Nagarajan, R., Keller, M. A., Kumar, R., Nielsen-Saines, K., Michalik, D. E., … Thomas, M. A. (2014). Regional brain gray and white matter changes in perinatally HIV-Infected adolescents. *NeuroImage: Clinical*, *4*, 29–34. https://doi.org/10.1016/j.nicl.2013.10.012

Senn, T. E., Carey, M. P., & Vanable, P. A. (2008). Childhood and adolescent sexual abuse and subsequent sexual risk behavior: Evidence from controlled studies, methodological critique, and suggestions for research. *Clinical Psychology Review*, *28*(5), 711–735. https://doi.org/10.1016/j.cpr.2007.10.002

Shoko, C., & Chikobvu, D. (2019). A superiority of viral load over CD4 cell count when predicting mortality in HIV patients on therapy. *BMC Infectious Diseases*, *19*(1), 1–10. https://doi.org/10.1186/s12879-019-3781-1

Shuttleworth-Edwards, A. B., Kemp, R. D., Rust, A. L., Muirhead, J. G. L., Hartman, N. P., & Radloff, S. E. (2004). Cross-cultural effects on IQ test performance: A review and preliminary normative indications on WAIS-III test performance. *Journal of Clinical and Experimental Neuropsychology*, *26*(7), 903–920. https://doi.org/10.1080/13803390490510824

Shuttleworth-Edwards, A. B., Van der Merwe, A. S., van Tonder, P., & Radloff, S. E. (2013). WISC-IV test performance in the South African context: A collation of cross-cultural norms. In *Psychological Assessment in South Africa: Research and Applications* 2000-2010. DOI./10.18772/22013015782.8

Shuttleworth-Jordan, A. B. (1996). On not reinventing the wheel: A clinical perspective on culturally relevant test usage in South Africa. *South African Journal of Psychology*, *26*(2), 96–102.

Shuttleworth-Jordan, A.B. & Bode, S.G. (1995). Use of the SAWAIS Digit Symbol Incidental Recall Test. *South African Journal of Psychology*, *25*, 53-57.

Smith, R., Chernoff, M., Williams, P. L., Malee, K. M., Sirois, P. A., Kammerer, B., … Rutstein, R. (2012). Impact of HIV severity on cognitive and adaptive functioning during childhood and adolescence. *Pediatric Infectious Disease Journal*, *31*(6), 592–598. https://doi.org/10.1097/INF.0b013e318253844b

Smith, R., & Wilkins, M. (2015). Perinatally acquired HIV infection: Long-term neuropsychological consequences and challenges ahead. *Child Neuropsychology*, *21*(2), 234–268. https://doi.org/10.1080/09297049.2014.898744

Solomon, T. M., & Halkitis, P. N. (2008). Cognitive executive functioning in relation to HIV medication adherence among gay, bisexual, and other men who have sex with men. *AIDS and Behavior*. https://doi.org/10.1007/s10461-007-9273-0

Spies, G., Ahmed-Leitao, F., Fennema-Notestine, C., Cherner, M., & Seedat, S. (2016). Effects of HIV and childhood trauma on brain morphometry and neurocognitive function. *Journal of NeuroVirology*, *22*(2), 149–158. https://doi.org/10.1007/s13365-015-0379-2

Statistics South Africa. (2019). Mid-year Population estimates. Retrieved from http://www.statssa.gov.sa

Statistics South Africa. (2018). Annual population estimates. Retrieved from http://www.statssa.gov.sa

Steinberg, L. (2005). Cognitive and affective development in adolescence. *Trends in Cognitive Sciences*, *9*(2), 69–74. https://doi.org/10.1016/j.tics.2004.12.005

Tan, I. L., & McArthur, J. C. (2012). HIV-associated neurological disorders: A guide to pharmacotherapy. *CNS Drugs*. https://doi.org/10.2165/11597770-000000000-00000

UNAIDS. (2018). Global report. Retrieved from http54s://www.unaids.org/sites/default/files/media_asset/unaids-data-2018_en.pdf

Tan, X., & Michel, R. (2011). Why do standardized testing programs report scaled scores. *ETS R & D Connections*, *16*, 1-6.

Van Rie, A., Harrington, P. R., Dow, A., & Robertson, K. (2007). Neurologic and neurodevelopmental manifestations of pediatric HIV/AIDS: A global perspective. *European Journal of Paediatric Neurology*, *11*(1), 1–9. https://doi.org/10.1016/j.ejpn.2006.10.006

Vanable, P. A., Carey, M. P., Brown, J. L., DiClemente, R. J., Salazar, L. F., Brown, L. K., … Stanton, B. F. (2009). Test-Retest Reliability of Self-Reported HIV/STD-Related Measures Among African-American Adolescents in Four U.S. Cities. *Journal of Adolescent Health*, *44*(3), 214–221. https://doi.org/10.1016/j.jadohealth.2008.09.002

Waldrop-Valverde, D., Jones, D. L., Gould, F., Kumar, M., & Ownby, R. L. (2010). Neurocognition, health-related reading literacy, and numeracy in medication management for HIV infection. *AIDS Patient Care and STDs*, *24*(8), 477–484. https://doi.org/10.1089/apc.2009.0300

Wechsler, D. (1999). Manual for the Wechsler abbreviated intelligence scale (WASI). In *WASI*.

Wechsler, David. (2003). Wechsler Intelligence Scale for Children-IV Conceptual and Interpretive Guide. *Indiana University - Purdue University Indianapolis*.

Wiener, L., Mellins, C. A., Marhefka, S., & Battles, H. B. (2007). Disclosure of an HIV diagnosis to children: History, current research, and future directions. *Journal of Developmental and Behavioral Pediatrics*. https://doi.org/10.1097/01.DBP.0000267570.87564.cd

Willen, E. J., Cuadra, A., Arheart, K. L., Post, M. J. D., & Govind, V. (2017). Young adults perinatally infected with HIV perform more poorly on measures of executive functioning and motor speed than ethnically matched healthy controls. *AIDS Care -*

Psychological and Socio-Medical Aspects of AIDS/HIV. https://doi.org/10.1080/09540121.2016.1234677

Williams, P. L., Storm, D., Montepiedra, G., Nichols, S., Kammerer, B., Sirois, P. A., … Malee, K. (2006). Predictors of adherence to antiretroviral medications in children and adolescents with HIV infection. *Pediatrics*, *118*(6). https://doi.org/10.1542/peds.2006-0493

Wood, S. M., Shah, S. S., Steenhoff, A. P., & Rutstein, R. M. (2009). The impact of AIDS diagnoses on long-term neurocognitive and psychiatric outcomes of surviving adolescents with perinatally acquired HIV. *AIDS*, *23*(14), 1859–1865. https://doi.org/10.1097/QAD.0b013e32832d924f

Woods, S. P., Moore, D. J., Weber, E., & Grant, I. (2009). Cognitive neuropsychology of HIV-associated neurocognitive disorders. *Neuropsychology Review*. https://doi.org/10.1007/s11065-009-9102-5

World Health Organization. (2010). Antiretroviral therapy for HIV infection in adults and adolescents: recommendations for a public health approach-2010 revision. https://apps.who.int/iris/bitstream/handle/10665/44379/9789241599764_eng.pdf (Accessed 31/10/2019)

World Health Organisation. (2019). HIV/AIDS. Retrieved from https://www.who.int/news-room/fact-sheets/detail/hiv-aids

World Health Organisation (2018). Maternal, new born, child and adolescent health. Retrieved from https://www.who.int/maternal_child_adolescent/topics/adolescence/second-decade/en/

Zillmer, E. a, Spiers, M. V, & Culbertson, W. C. (2008). Principles of neuropsychology. Belmont, CA: Thomson Wadsworth.

APPENDIX A

Paediatric Neuropsychology Development Questionnaire (PNDQ)_Short Form

Child's Name: ______________________________ Date of Birth: ___________________Age: _________

PREGNANCY AND BIRTH

Were there any complications during the *pregnancy*?

Did you take any medicine during pregnancy? Prescribed or over the counter?

Did you smoke cigarettes while you were pregnant? If so, how many?

Did you drink when you were pregnant? If so, how much?

Anything else, like dagga? Any drugs?

Was the birth on time?

If early or late, find out why

Was it a natural birth or via C-section/Caesarian? Was labor induced?

Were there any complications during the birth?

Were there any early *separations* from you? (when and for how long)

Have there been any *emotionally difficult* experiences for your child?

SCHOOLING

What *type* of school does your child attend? (mainstream / special needs)

Has your child repeated any Grades?

MEDICAL / MENTAL HEALTH

Has your child ever been referred to a *Psychologist/Psychiatry* service?

Please give any details of any medical or *mental health problems* you, your child, or your family of origin may have had/have.

What *medication* is your child currently receiving?

Name of History-Taker: ___________________________ Date: __________ Signed: _______________

APPENDIX B

Adolescent/Caregiver Consent Form

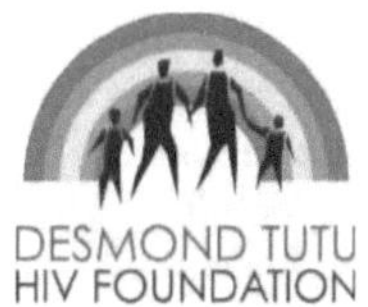

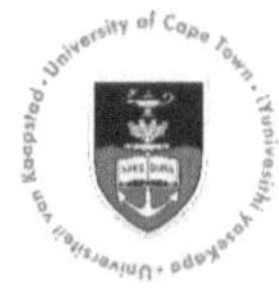

"Retaining HIV-positive youth in care: A model for transitioning adolescents receiving ART from paediatric to adult care" - Aim 1 Adolescent Parent/Caregiver Consent Form

Short title: HlangananiPlus HCT

Introduction

We are doing research in order to understand whether a youth programme that prepares youth to move from adolescent care to adult care including information around health education, communication and life skills, goal management, information about treatment and treatment adherence (commitment to taking treatment regularly) will help prepare the youth better when they are moved to the adult clinic. As you know, as youth get older, they will need to be moved to the adult clinic and will begin to receive their treatment and other health services thereon. We want to see if having a programme like this will help ease this process for your child as compared to the usual standard of care.

What is my child being asked to do? We are asking your child to be in a research study that will help us find out more about whether people his/her age will benefit from such a program, so that when they move, they are able to come to their regular appointments, continue coming to the clinic and take their treatment regularly and as discussed with their doctor. We ask you to fully read this form or have it read to you to decide if you want your child to join the study. Please ask if there is anything that is not clear or if you would like more information.

Why is my child being asked to help? We are asking you to help with this research because your child is between 14 and 24 years of age. One of the groups of people participating in the research is adolescents.

How many people are expected to participate in the research? 120 participants will be included this part of the study. They will be randomly put into two groups with 60 people in each group. One group will participate in the program and the other will receive the standard (usual) care at the Hannan Crusaid clinic in Gugulethu. Your child has been assigned to the group that will participate in the program.

Does my child have to take part? Not at all. You can decide that your child should not be included in the research. If you are unsure, you can make the decision about your child being in the research later by using the information included in this form and talking to our research staff. If you do decide that your child will take part in this research, we will ask you to sign this form as a sign that you understand this information and that you agree for your child to be in the research. You will get a copy of the form to keep. Even if you agree for your child to be in the study now by signing this form, you can still change your mind at any time and withdraw your child from the study.

What will be done if my child takes part in this research study? If you agree for your child to participate in this study by signing this form, the interviewer will sit down with your child and ask him/her questions. The interviewer will begin by introducing and giving your child more details about the programme. Then they will ask your child questions about their background like school, age and gender. They will also ask your child about people he/she lives with at home, about his/her parents or care givers, whether they work or not. We will ask your child about knowledge of HIV and AIDS as well as their knowledge of treatment. This discussion will take roughly 30 minutes.

Second, your child will be asked to complete some games (e.g., problem solving and memory games) and puzzles tests to see whether he/she needs further help when it comes to treatment adherence. The whole process will take about 2 hours. You can stop if you are feeling tired and need to take a break, at any time.

Third, your child might be requested to take part in-depth interviews where the researcher will ask him/her more questions about their life history, about their parents, about their disclosure process. They will also ask your child about community perceptions of HIV, history of ARV treatment and adherence, barriers to and facilitators of treatment adherence, feelings around living with HIV, and their future plans.

Fourth, your child will be asked to come for sessions every week for 17 weeks, which will be held every Saturday at the scout hall near the Hannan clinic. During these sessions, that is when our training and activities will take place.

What if the questions upset my child? If your child feels uncomfortable answering any of the questions on the survey, he/ she does not have to answer. He/she will be able to stop being in the study at any time. Also, we have a counselor who will be working with us and if you are upset and need more assistance, the counselor will be there to assist you.

Does you child get paid to be a part of this study? You will be not be paid for being in the study but we will pay your child's transport of R30 every time we meet for our sessions. Your child will also receive a meal after the session for lunch.

Will what my child says be kept confidential? Yes. All the information that is given to us will be kept confidential (private). Anonymity (your name and other details being unknown) and confidentiality is a high priority and every effort will be made to protect it. The information collected will be secured, locked and/or password-protected within the DTHC offices. To safe guard against any loss, the recording of your interview will be stored on a safe and secure online facility called shared-point that allows access of your interview to only staff members working on this project. A backup will be stored on only one computer that is protected by a password at our head offices. We will not use actual names, but instead use a number identification system to distinguish between participants. If the results of this research are published or presented, your name will not be included in the study.

Who should I contact for further information? If you have questions about the study, you can call the principal investigator, Millicent Atujuna, at 021 406 6961.

Who can I call for information about my child's rights as someone who is helping with research?
There is a group of doctors and researchers whose job it is to help see that research is done carefully and that people in the research are treated fairly and it is made as safe as possible. If you have any questions about these things, or if you have a complaint or complaints about your rights and wellbeing as a participant, please contact the Human Research Ethics Committee: Tel: 021 406 6492 E-mail: sumaya.ariefdien@uct.ac.za

STATEMENT OF CONSENT:

I have read the information about this study and understand the explanations of it that were verbally given to me. I have had my questions concerning the study answered and understand what will be required of my child if he/she takes part in this study.

You voluntarily consent to allow your child to participate in this study. You hereby authorize the collection, use and sharing of your child's performance and other data. By signing this form, you are not waiving any of your legal rights.

SIGNATURES

____ ____________________

Signature of Person Consenting and Authorizing Date

____ ____________________

Name of Child Age

__________________ __________________ ____________________

Study Staff Member Study Staff Member's Signature Date

Conducting IC Discussion (print)

____________________ __________________ _________________________

Witness' Name (print) Witness' Signature Date

NOTE: This form with the original signatures MUST be retained on file by the principal investigator. A copy must be given to the participant. A copy should be placed in the participant's medical record, if applicable.

APPENDIX C

Adolescent Assent Form

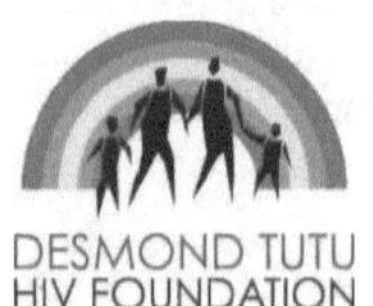

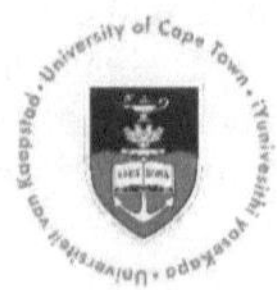

"Retaining HIV-positive youth in care: A model for transitioning adolescents receiving ART from paediatric to adult care" - Aim 1 Adolescent Assent Form

Short title: HlangananiPlus HCT

Note to research staff: Only adolescents who have provided you with a written parent or caregiver consent form can participate in the assent process. Parent or caregiver signatures should appear on the parent consent form.

Introduction

We are doing research in order to understand whether a youth programme that prepares youth to move from adolescent care to adult care including information around health education, communication and life skills, goal management, information about treatment and treatment adherence (commitment to taking treatment regularly) will help prepare the youth better when they are moved to the adult clinic. As you know, as youth get older, they will need to be moved to the adult clinic and will begin to receive their treatment and other health services thereon. We want to see if having a programme like this will help ease this process.

What am I being asked to do? We are asking you to be in a research study that will help us find out more about whether people your age will benefit from such a program so that when they move, they are able to come to their regular appointments, continue coming to the clinic and take their treatment regularly and as discussed with their doctor. We ask you to fully read this form or have it read to you to decide if you want to join the study. Please ask if there is anything that is not clear or if you would like more information.

Why am I being asked to help? We are asking you to help with this research because you are between 14 and 24 years of age. One of the groups of people participating in the research is adolescents.

How many people are expected to participate in the research? 120 participants will be included this part of the study. They will be randomly put into two groups with 60 people in each group. One group will participate in the program, and the other will receive the standard (usual) care at the Hannan Crusaid clinic in Gugulethu. You have been assigned to the group that will participate in the program.

Do I have to take part? Not at all. You can decide to not to be included in the research. If you are unsure, you can make the decision about being in the research by using the information included in this form and talking to our research staff. If you do decide to be in the research, we will ask you to sign this form as a sign that you understand this information and that you agree to be in the research. You will get a copy of the form to keep. Even if you agree to be in the study now by signing this form, you can still change your mind at any time and withdraw from the study.

What will be done if you take part in this research study? If you agree to participate in this study by signing this form, the interviewer will sit down with you and ask you questions. The interviewer will begin by introducing and giving you more details about the programme. Then they will ask you questions about your background like school, age and gender. They will also ask you about people you live with at home, about your parents or your care givers, whether they work or not. We will ask you about knowledge of HIV and AIDS as well as your knowledge of treatment. This discussion will take roughly 30 minutes.

Second, you will be asked to complete some games (e.g., problem solving and memory games) and puzzles, tests to see whether you need further help when it comes to treatment adherence. The whole process will take about 2 hours. You can stop if you are feeling tired and need to take a break, at any time.

Third, you might be requested to take part in-depth interviews where the researcher will ask you more questions about your life history, about your parents, about your disclosure process. They will also ask you about community perceptions of HIV, history of ARV treatment and adherence, barriers to and facilitators of treatment adherence, feelings around living with HIV, and your future plans.

Fourth, you will be asked to come for sessions every week, for 17 weeks, which will be held every Saturday at the scout hall near the Hannan clinic. During these sessions, that is when our training and activities will take place.

What if the questions upset me? If you feel uncomfortable answering any of the questions on the survey, you will still be able to stop being in the study at any time. Also, we have a counselor who will be working with us and if you are upset and need more assistance, the counselor will be there to assist you.

Do I get paid to be a part of this study? You will be not be paid for being in the study but we will pay your transport of R30 every time we meet for our sessions. You will also receive a meal after the session for lunch.

Will what I say be kept confidential? Yes. All the information that is given to us will be kept confidential (private). Anonymity (your name and other details being unknown) and confidentiality is a high priority and every effort will be made to protect it. The information collected will be secured, locked and/or password-protected within the DTHC offices. To safe guard against any loss, the recording of your interview will be stored on a safe and secure online facility called shared-point that allows access of your interview to only staff members working on this project. A backup will be stored on only one computer that is protected by a password at our head offices. We will not use actual names, but instead use a number identification system to distinguish between participants. If the results of this research are published or presented, your name will not be included in the study.

Who should I contact for further information? If you have questions about the study, you can call the principal investigator, Millicent Atujuna, at 021 406 6961.

Who can I call for information about my rights as someone who is helping with research?

There is a group of doctors and researchers whose job it is to help see that research is done carefully and that people in the research are treated fairly and it is made as safe as possible. If you have any questions about these things, or if you have a complaint or complaints about your rights and wellbeing as a research participant, please contact the Human Research Ethics Committee: Tel: 021 406 6492 E-mail: sumaya.ariefdien@uct.ac.za

STATEMENT OF CONSENT:

I have read the information about this study and understand the explanations of it that were verbally given to me. I have had my questions concerning the study answered and understand what will be required of me if I take part in this study.

SIGNATURES

____________________	____________________	____________________
Volunteer's Name (print)	Volunteer's Signature	Date

____________________	____________________	__________
Study Staff Member Conducting IC Discussion (print)	Study Staff Member's Signature	Date

____________________	____________________	____________________
Witness' Name (print)	Witness' Signature	Date

NOTE: This form with the original signatures MUST be retained on file by the principal investigator. A copy must be given to the participant. A copy should be placed in the participant's medical record, if applicable.

APPENDIX D

Adolescent Parent/Caregiver Control Consent Form

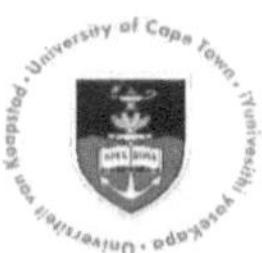

"The executive function outcomes associated with HIV-positive adolescents in South Africa" - Adolescent Parent/Caregiver Control Consent Form

Introduction

We are doing research in order to determine whether there are significant executive function (e.g., thinking, planning and flexibility) differences between HIV-positive adolescents and HIV-negative adolescents.

What is my child being asked to do? We are asking your child to be in a research study that will help us find out more about whether people his/her age differ from those who are HIV-positive when performing a variety of cognitive tasks. We ask you to fully read this form or have it read to you to decide if you want your child to join the study. Please ask if there is anything that is not clear or if you would like more information.

Why is my child being asked to help? We are asking your child to help with this research because your child is HIV-negative and between 14 and 16 years of age.

How many people are expected to participate in the research? 60 participants will be included in this part of the study. One group of 30 will be HIV-positive, and the remaining 30 will be HIV negative. Your child has been asked to be a part of the HIV negative group.

Does my child have to take part? Not at all. You can decide that you child should not to be included in the research. If you are unsure, you can make the decision about your child being in the research by using the information included in this form and talking to our research staff. If you do decide that your child will take part in this research, we will ask you to sign this form as a sign that you understand this information and that you agree for your child to be in the research. You will get a copy of the form to keep. Even if you agree for your child to be in the study now by signing this form, you can still change your mind at any time and withdraw your child from the study.

What will be done if my child takes part in this research study? If you agree for your child to participate in this study by signing this form, the interviewer will sit down with your child and ask him/her questions. The interviewer will begin by introducing and giving your child more details about the study. Then they will ask your child questions about their background like school, age and gender. They will also ask your child about people he/she lives with at home, about his/her parents or care givers, whether they work or not. This discussion will take roughly 30 minutes.

Second, your child will be asked to complete some games (e.g., problem solving and memory games) and puzzles tests. The whole process will take about 2 hours. Your child can stop if they are feeling tired and need to take a break, at any time.

What if the questions upset my child? If your child feels uncomfortable answering any of the questions on the survey, he/ she does not have to answer. He/she will be able to stop being in the study at any time. Also, we have a counselor who will be working with us and if your child or you are upset and need more assistance, the counselor will be there to assist them.

Does your child get paid to be a part of this study? Your child will be not be paid for being in the study but we will pay your child's transport of R30 on the day he/she comes in for testing if he/she has to travel to the testing venue. Your child will also receive a R50 meal voucher after testing for lunch.

Will what my child says be kept confidential? Yes. All the information that is given to us will be kept confidential (private). Anonymity (your child's name and other details being unknown) and confidentiality is a high priority and every effort will be made to protect it. The information collected will be secured, locked and/or password-protected within the Department of Psychology at the University of Cape Town. We will not use actual names, but instead use a number identification system to distinguish between participants. If the results of this research are published or presented, your child's name will not be included in the study.

Who should I contact for further information? If you have questions about the study, you

can call the principal investigator, Bryony Dyssell, on 072 232 7862 and Vakele Gama on 0738307778.

Who can I call for information about my child's rights as someone who is helping with research?

There is a group of researchers whose job it is to help see that research is done

carefully and that people in the research are treated fairly and it is made as safe as possible.

If you have any questions about these things, or if you have a complaint or complaints about your rights and well-being as a participant, please contact the Department of Psychology Research Ethics Committee: Tel: 021 650 4104

E-mail: rosalind.adams@uct.ac.za

STATEMENT OF CONSENT:

I have read the information about this study and understand the explanations of it that were verbally given to me. I have had my questions concerning the study answered and understand what will be required of my child if he/she takes part in this study.

You voluntarily consent to allow your child to participate in this study. You hereby authorize the collection, use and sharing of your child's performance and other data. By signing this form, you are not waiving any of your legal rights.

SIGNATURES

____ ____________________

Signature of Person Consenting and Authorizing Date

____ ____________________

Name of Child Age

__________________ __________________ ____________________

Study Staff Member Study Staff Member's Signature Date

Conducting IC Discussion (print)

____________________ __________________ _________________________

Witness' Name (print) Witness' Signature Date

NOTE: This form with the original signatures MUST be retained on file by the principal investigator. A copy must be given to the participant. A copy should be placed in the participant's medical record, if applicable.

APPENDIX E

Adolescent Control Assent Form

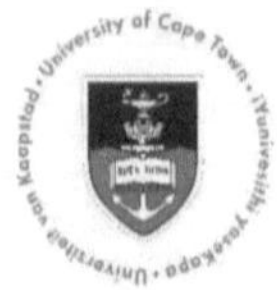

"The executive function outcomes associated with HIV-positive adolescents in South Africa" - Adolescent Control Assent Form

Note to research staff: Only adolescents who have provided you with a written parent or caregiver consent form can participate in the assent process. Parent or caregiver signatures should appear on the parent consent form.

Introduction

We are doing research in order to determine whether there are significant executive function (e.g., thinking, planning and flexibility) differences between HIV-positive adolescents and HIV-negative adolescents.

What am I being asked to do? We are asking you to be in a research study that will help us find out more about whether people your age differ from those who are HIV-positive when performing a variety of cognitive tasks. We ask you to fully read this form or have it read to you to decide if you want to join the study. Please ask if there is anything that is not clear or if you would like more information.

Why am I being asked to help? We are asking you to help with this research because you are HIV-negative and between 14 and 16 years of age.

How many people are expected to participate in the research? 60 participants will be included in this study. One group of 30 will be HIV-positive, and the remaining 30 will be HIV negative. You have been asked to be a part of the HIV negative group.

Do I have to take part? Not at all. You can decide not to be included in the research. If you are unsure, you can make the decision about being in the research by using the information included in this form and talking to our research staff. If you do decide to be in the research, we will ask you to sign this form as a sign that you understand this information and that you agree to be in the research. You will get a copy of the form to keep. Even if you agree to be in the study now by signing this form, you can still change your mind at any time and withdraw from the study.

What will be done if you take part in this research study? If you agree to participate in this study by signing this form, the interviewer will sit down with you and ask you questions. The interviewer will begin by introducing and giving you more details about the study. Then they will ask you questions about your background like school, age and gender. They will also ask you about people you live with at home, about your parents or care givers, whether they work or not. This discussion will take roughly 30 minutes.

Second, you will be asked to complete some games (e.g., problem solving and memory games) and puzzle tests. The whole process will take about 2 hours. You can stop if you are feeling tired and need to take a break, at any time.

What if the questions upset me? If you feel uncomfortable answering any of the questions on the survey, you will still be able to stop being in the study at any time. Also, we have a counselor who will be working with us and if you are upset and need more assistance, the counselor will be there to assist you.

Do I get paid to be a part of this study? You will not be paid for being in the study but we will pay your transport of R30 on the day you come in for testing if you need to travel to the testing venue. You will also receive a R50 meal voucher after testing for lunch.

Will what I say be kept confidential? Yes. All the information that is given to us will be kept confidential (private). Anonymity (your name and other details being unknown) and confidentiality is a high priority and every effort will be made to protect it. The information collected will be secured, locked and/or password-protected within the Department of Psychology at the University of Cape Town. We will not use actual names, but instead use a number identification system to distinguish between participants. If the results of this research are published or presented, your name will not be included in the study.

Who should I contact for further information? If you have questions about the study, you

can call the principal investigator, Bryony Dyssell, on 072 232 7862 and Vakele Gama at 0738307778

Who can I call for information about my rights as someone who is helping with research?

There is a group of researchers whose job it is to help see that research is done

carefully and that people in the research are treated fairly and it is made as safe as possible.

If you have any questions about these things, or if you have a complaint or complaints about

your rights and well-being as a research participant, please contact the Department of Psychology Research Ethics Committee: Tel: 021 650 4104,

E-mail: rosalind.adams@uct.ac.za

STATEMENT OF CONSENT:

I have read the information about this study and understand the explanations of it that were verbally given to me. I have had my questions concerning the study answered and understand what will be required of me if I take part in this study.

SIGNATURES

____________________	____________________	____________________
Volunteer's Name (print)	Volunteer's Signature	Date

____________________	____________________	____________________
Study Staff Member Conducting IC Discussion (print)	Study Staff Member's Signature	Date

____________________	____________________	____________________
Witness' Name (print)	Witness' Signature	Date

NOTE: This form with the original signatures MUST be retained on file by the principal investigator. A copy must be given to the participant. A copy should be placed in the participant's medical record, if applicable.

APPENDIX F

Test Order

1. Numbers
2. Sky Search
3. WASI
4. Inhibition
5. Coding
6. Symbol Search
7. CCTT
8. Verbal fluency
9. Towers

APPENDIX G

Ethical Clearance HlangananiPlus

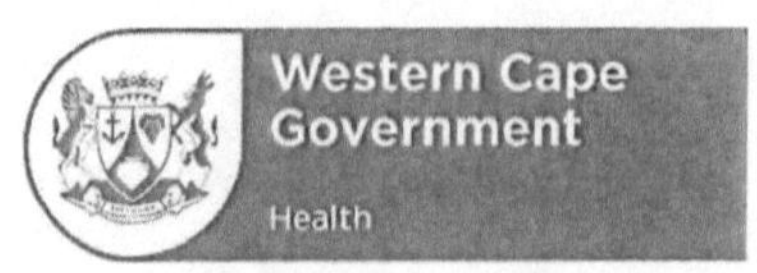

HEALTH IMPACT ASSESSMENT HEALTH RESEARCH SUB DIRECTORATE Health Research@westerncape.gov.za tel: +27 21 483 0866: fax: +27 21 483 9895 5th Floor, Norton Rose House,, 8 Riebeek Street, Cape Town, 8001 vvwvv.capegateway .gov .za)

REFERENCE: WC 201711 003 ENQUIRIES:

ES: Dr Sabela Petros

Dr Sabela Petros

University of Cape Town

Anzio Road

Observatory

Cape Town

7925

For attention: Dr Millicent Atujuna

Re: Retaining HIV-positive youth in care: A model for transitioning adolescents receiving ART from

paediatric to adult care: HlcngananiPlus.

Thank you for submitting your proposal to undertake the above-mentioned study. We are pleased

to inform you that the department has granted you approval for your research. Please contact

following people to assist you with any further enquiries in accessing the following sites:

Gugulethu CHC	Mr Lunga Makamba	021 633 0020

Kindly ensure that the following are adhered to:

1. Arrangements can be made with managers, providing that normal activities at requested

facilities are not interrupted.

2. Researchers, in accessing provincial health facilities, are expressing consent to provide the

   department with an electronic copy of the final feedback (annexure 9) within six months of

   completion of research. This can be submitted to the provincial Research Co-ordinator

   (Health.Research@westerncape.gov.za).

3. In the event where the research project goes beyond the estimated completion date

which was submitted, researchers are expected to complete and submit a progress report (Annexure 8) to the provincial Research Co-ordinator

(Health.Research@westerncape.gov.za).

4. The reference number above should be quoted in all future correspondence.

Yours sincerely

AJ HAWKRIDGE

WKRIDGE

DR A HAW RIDG DIRECTOR: HEALTH IMPACT ASSESSMENT

DATE: 1 7- // 2017 cc: P OLCKERS DIRECTOR: KLIPFONTEIN/ MITCHELLS PLAIN

APPENDIX H

Ethical Clearance Department of Psychology

UNIVERSITY OF CAPE TOWN

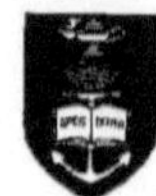

Department of Psychology

University of Cape Town Rondebosch 7701 South Africa
Telephone (021) 650 3417
Fax No. (021) 650 4104

07 March 2017

Vakele Gama
Department of Psychology
University of Cape Town
Rondebosch 7701

Dear Vakele

I am pleased to inform you that ethical clearance has been given by an Ethics Review Committee of the Faculty of Humanities for your study, Investigating the efficacy of a Goal Management Training (GMT) intervention in increasing adherence to antiretroviral therapy among adolescents living with HIV in South Africa. (The title for the larger study, which it forms a part of, is: Retaining HIV-positive youth in care: A model for transitioning adolescents receiving ART from pediatric to adult care (HCT)). The reference number is PSY2017-003.

I wish you all the best for your study.

Yours sincerely

Lauren Wild (PhD)
Associate Professor
Chair: Ethics Review Committee

University of Cape Town
ΨPSYCHOLOGY DEPARTMENT
Upper Campus
Rondebosch

APPENDIX I

Revised Ethical Clearance Department of Psychology

UNIVERSITY OF CAPE TOWN

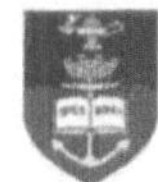

Department of Psychology

University of Cape Town Rondebosch 7701 South Africa
Telephone (021) 650 3417
Fax No. (021) 650 4104

15 August 2018

Ms Bryony Dyssell
Department of Psychology
University of Cape Town
Rondebosch 7701

Dear Ms Dyssell

I am pleased to inform you that ethical clearance has been given by an Ethics Review Committee of the Faculty of Humanities for the amended protocol, submitted 15 August 2018, to your study, *The executive function outcomes associated with HIV-positive adolescents in South Africa.* The reference number remains PSY2018-032.

I wish you all the best for your study.

Yours sincerely,

Lauren Wild (PhD)
Associate Professor
Chair: Ethics Review Committee

APPENDIX J

Qualitative Description of WASI Scaled Scores

Qualitative Descriptions of WASI Scores

IQ Scores	Sub-test scaled score	Classification
130 and above	16 -19	Very superior
120 - 129	14-15	Superior
110 - 119	12 -13	High Average
90 – 109	8 – 11	Average
80 – 89	6 – 7	Low Average
70 – 79	4 – 5	Borderline
69 and below	1 - 3	Extremely Low

Note. Taken from Wechler Abbreviated Scale of Intelligence (Wechsler, 1999)

APPENDIX K

TABLE 6 *Neuropsychological Variables: Between-Group Comparisons*

	HIV group (n = 22)				Control group (n = 22)				Test Statistics		
Variable (scaled scores)	*n*	*M (SD)*	*Median*	*Range*	*n*	*M (SD)*	*Median*	*Range*	*t*	*p*	ESE
Cognitive Flexibility											
Numbers Backwards	22	5.55 (2.92)	5.00	2-15	22	6.82 (3.52)	7.00	13	1.30	.100	0.39
Switching Combined	20	4.35 (2.80)	4.00	1-12	22	5.23 (2.88)	5.00	11	1.00	.162	0.31
Verbal Fluency Condition 3	22	5.82 (3.20)	6.00	1-19	22	7.32 (4.26)	6.50	18	1.32	.097	0.40
Verbal Fluency Switching accuracy	22	3.50 (1.60)	4.00	1-9	22	3.95 (2.01)	3.50	8	0.83	.206	0.25
Children's Colour trails test 2	22	65.32 (44.32)	53.50	28-81	22	52.14 (13.86)	52.50	53	-1.33	.095	0.40
Information Processing											
Coding	22	4.68 (2.19)	4.00	1-10	22	5.50 (2.22)	5.50	9	1.23	.128	0.37
Symbol Search	22	6.82 (2.94)	7.00	1-14	22	7.77 (3.53)	7.50	13	0.98	.168	0.29
Verbal Fluency: Condition 1	22	4.73 (3.04)	4.50	1-10	22	6.09 (2.49)	6.00	9	1.63	.055	0.49
Verbal Fluency: Condition 2	21	6.76 (3.06)	6.00	2-16	22	7.82 (3.74)	7.00	14	1.01	.159	0.31
Attentional Control											
Inhibition Combined	22	5.00(3.63)	5.00	1-11	22	5.64 (2.87)	6.00	10	0.65	.261	0.20
Inhibition Total Errors	22	3.00 (2.62)	1.00	1-13	22	4.05 (3.43)	3.50	12	1.14	.131	0.34
Goal Setting											
Similarities	22	4.23 (3.10)	3.00	1-10	22	5.23 (3.07)	5.50	9	1.08	.144	0.32
Matrix Reasoning	22	4.95 (2.94)	5.00	1-10	22	4.36 (2.68)	4.00	9	-0.70	.245	0.21
Tower: Achievement score	22	8.36 (2.34)	9.00	4-13	22	9.05 (2.24)	9.00	9	0.99	.165	0.30
Tower: Time move ratio	22	10.50 (2.06)	11.00	5-13	22	10.32 (2.28)	11.00	8	-0.28	.392	0.08

Tower: Rules violations ratio	22	9.00 (2.25)	10.00	1-10	22	8.86 (2.70)	10.00	9	-0.18	.428	0.06
Towers: Move accuracy	22	7.95 (2.57)	8.00	2-11	22	7.45 (2.70)	8.00	9	-0.63	.267	0.19

Note: p-values are one-tailed

APPENDIX L

Boxplots Showing Outliers

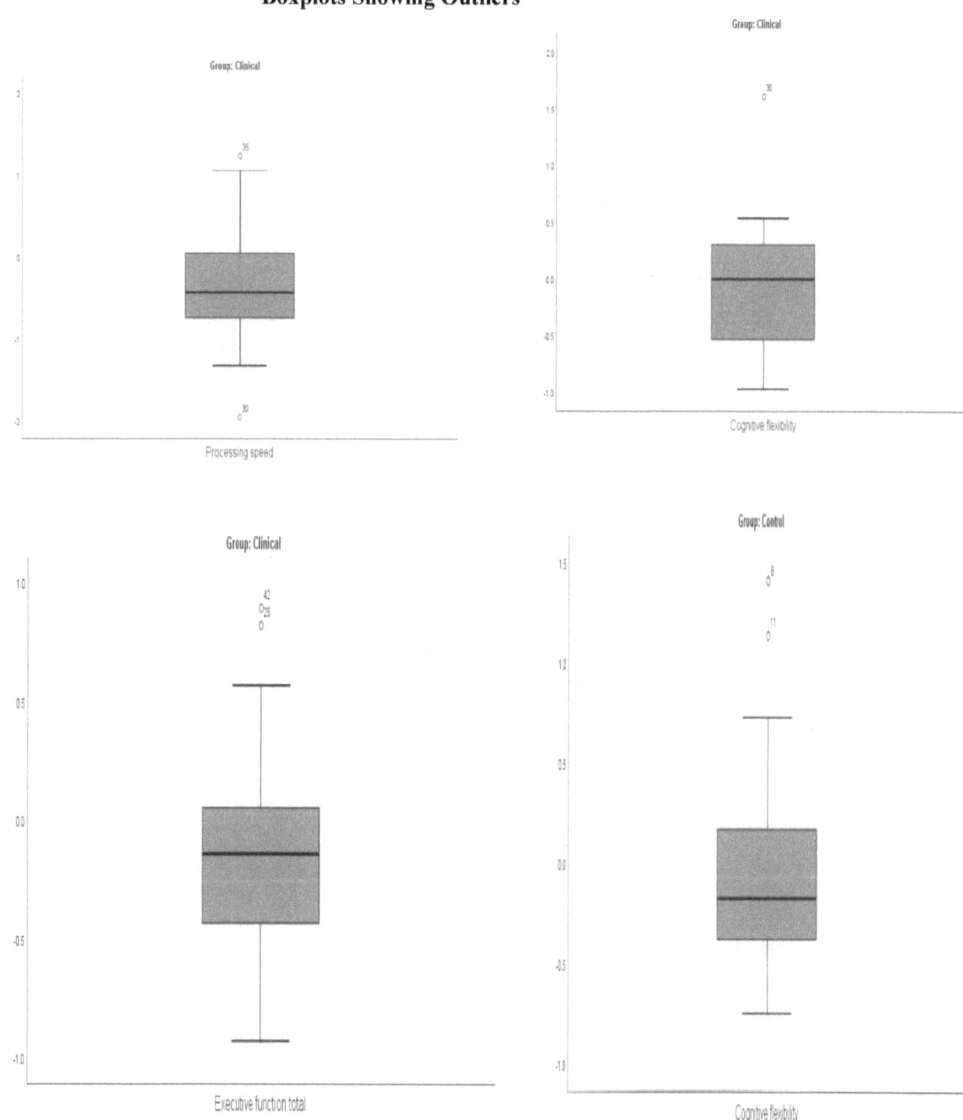

Note: Clinical group refers to HIV-positive group, Control group refers to HIV-negative group

APPENDIX M

PROJECT LEADER/PRINCIPAL INVESTIGATORS	
Name: Millicent Atujuna,PhD Organization: Desmond Tutu HIV Centre Address: University of Cape Town Werner and Biet Building North Anzio Road, Mowbray Cape Town 7925	Tel: +27 21 406 6961 Mobile: +27 825187551 Fax: +27 21 650 6963 E-mail: Millicent.atujuna@hiv-research.org.za
PROJECT CO INVESTIGATORS	
Name: Prof. Linda-Gail Bekker, MBChB, FCP(SA), PhD Organization: Desmond Tutu HIV Centre Address: University of Cape Town Werner and Biet Building North Anzio Road, Mowbray Cape Town 7925	Tel: +27 21 650 6959 Mobile: +27 83 266 2876 Fax: +27 21 650 6963 E-mail: linda-gail.bekker@hiv-research.org.za
Name: Tiarney D.Ritchwood, PhD Organization: Desmond Tutu HIV Centre Address: University of Cape Town Werner and Biet Building North Anzio Road, Mowbray Cape Town 7925	Tel: +27 21 650 6959 Fax: +27 21 650 6963 E-mail: tiarney.ritchwood@hiv-research.org.za
Name: Rebecca Marcus, MBChB Organization: Desmond Tutu HIV Centre Address: University of Cape Town Werner and Biet Building North Anzio Road, Mowbray Cape Town 7925	Tel: +27 21 650 6959 Fax: +27 21 650 6963 E-mail: Rebecca.marcus@hiv-research.org.za
PROJECT COORDINATOR	
Name: Sheily Busiswe Ndwayana Organization: Desmond Tutu HIV Centre Address: University of Cape Town Werner and Biet Building North Anzio Road, Mowbray Cape Town 7925	Tel: +27 21 406 6961 Mobile: +27 834777642 Fax: +27 21 650 6963 E-mail: sheily.ndwayana@hiv-research.org.za

APPENDIX N Details of Translators

Name of Translator	Training Formal/ Informal	Previous Clinical Translation work
Minah Koela	Formal	• Translator at the Red Cross War Memorial Hospital at the Paediatric Neuropsychological Clinic • Translator at UCT Paarl Lung and Health study
Thozama Madze	Formal	• Translator at UCT Paarl Lung and Health study
Limpho Mokoena	Informal	• Translator at the Red Cross War Memorial Hospital at the Paediatric Neuropsychological Clinic • Translator at the Groote Schuur Adult Neuropsychological Clinic

www.ingramcontent.com/pod-product-compliance
Lightning Source LLC
LaVergne TN
LVHW041459190726
843491LV00008B/2439